Towards a Psychosomatic Conception
of Hypochondria

Martine Derzelle

Towards a Psychosomatic Conception of Hypochondria

The Impeded Thought

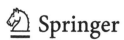 Springer

Martine Derzelle
Institut Jean-Godinot
Reims
France

ISBN 978-3-319-37976-0   ISBN 978-3-319-03053-1   (eBook)
DOI 10.1007/978-3-319-03053-1
Springer Cham Heidelberg New York Dordrecht London

Printed on acid-free paper

Springer is part of Springer Science+Business Media (www.springer.com)

Foreword

What a surprising title! "The Impeded Thought." But by whom? By what? An external censorship imposing a norm that replaces reality? An internal censorship confused with the norm it strives to recreate? Asking such questions about a concept like hypochondria suggests the uncommon liberty of an unfettered reflection, free to get to the heart of things: questioning itself as well as questioning its object. Extreme approach but only possible way to recognize that "obvious things," isolated from the objectification process that produced them, have become inescapable epistemological obstacles, and that, to go beyond the resulting locked-up thought, only a radical reflection on locked-up thought itself can help. This double motion exemplarily animates this work that simultaneously describes a closure, more and more totalizing, and an opening toward a counter-thinking which is also a thought of the object.

Why is this approach so complex?

Because the concept of hypochondria, which Freud said remained "a disgraceful lacuna" in the psychoanalytical edifice, has many times been used to justify proliferating theoretical constructs referring to the same energetic model. A model that considers hypochondria as an internal process caused by the fixation of anxiety, which is said to correspond to the direct transformation of libido, on to the affected part of the body. We then realize that this process has no end: whenever the hypochondriac is told that he has nothing, this "nothing" cannot put an end to his suffering, which is real; whenever his real suffering is recognized, its origin cannot be found. "Imaginary" perhaps, but still there, inscribed in the real body and defeating all therapeutic attempts. What is found here is an impasse that we really should define as relational, for organic complaint implies the other person's presence and decisive role.

Hypochondria thus seems to be an impasse-related pathology, as well as a psychosis and an organic pathology, consistent with a conception of psychosomatics that the author adopted and which posits that the most elementary psychosomatic phenomenon is not a process in itself, but a process linked to a conflict situation that may sometimes result in an impasse.

Henceforth, everything is clear: in hypochondria, therapeutic failure, instead of an accident, is the specific form taken by impasse in a pathology derived from impasse and that has to be thought as such. From what, for the first time, the possibility of appropriate therapeutic action emerges.

Thanks to the extreme care taken in its construction, whose every movement is associated with the pleasure of thinking, this book maliciously appears like a lasso whose formation we gradually follow until it is finally thrown to capture the object. And the thought that we have here does not close on itself, but provides an unhoped-for opening where thought and object freely develop, to consider, for instance, that the phenomenon of hypochondria, could be found outside of its association, developed here, with paranoia.

M. Sami-Ali

Acknowledgments

I am thankful to the "friends" who help me,
to the "villains" who stir my conscience...

I particularly thank Prof. Sami-Ali,

Prof. Albert Cattan,
Honorary Director of the Anti-Cancer Center of Reims,

Dr. Christian Pozzo di Borgo,
my partner at the Pain Consultation.

The headlong stream is termed violent,
but the river bed hemming it in is termed violent by no one.

Bertolt Brecht

Contents

Introduction

Abstract The study of hypochondria is likely to question theory and to generate fruitful conceptual developments. Justification.

Described many times but seldom questioned, diversely controversial but hardly explained, scandalously impossible to treat but little theorized, hypochondria is an enigma. Or rather an "uncannily familiar" notion. Obvious and questioning at the same time, combining overflowing extension and insufficient comprehension.

Obvious first. Ubiquitary syndrome as old as the medical speech itself, as it is one of its most ancient terms, identified by Hippocrates, named by Galen, hypochondria seems totally transparent, immediately understandable, subsumable within such a character as Molière's Argan, the Imaginary Invalid. Common-sense comprehension seems sufficient for its understanding, blindly sufficient thanks to its spatial and temporal proximity, in terms of "always" and "everywhere".

Question then. If, which is remarkable, hypochondria has hardly ever been precisely defined, its obviousness disappears as soon as you confront a patient whose whole life is filled with an essential complaint expressing "pain" and "belief that the body is affected". And when the conceptual frameworks of hysteria, depression, or delusion (Ford 1983, p.76 sq.) are invoked to locate this complaint, one cannot but notice the striking gap between the hypochondriacs on the one hand, and the hysterics, the depressed, and the delusional on the other hand.

Finally, consistent with its commonplace meaning which excessively simplifies the content of its clinical reality and turns it into an anonymous typical category— i.e., "imaginary illness"— hypochondria can only be given a status negatively, i.e., through what it helps avoiding: as a lack of elaboration, a defense against psychosis, an equivalent of depression. In short, everything that reinforces transparency, so that only something else can be seen through it, something that could have been and that is not.

Hypochondria: between a lack of definition and a definition through the lack, between a thought deficiency and a thought of deficiency. As if its obviousness prevented us from raising the real issues.

Can the double-centered paranoid schizophrenic, the paraphrenic who thinks his body is invaded by countless enemies, the melancholic denier, the doctor-persecuting paranoid, the "Argan"-like subject affected with hypochondriac "neurosis" be categorized under the same "label"? What distinguishes hypochondria as a problem? How can we think the resolution of the contradictions inherent to it as to the more general concept of actual neuroses? What positive content can be given to an entirely negative designation which is a reality created by a normative system of thought? There are many unresolved issues and they reveal a theoretical gap.

In this situation, resulting from an obstacle to thought which revives an old childhood tradition—preferring to veil one's eyes instead of admitting that the "sexual theory" is inaccurate—there are several possibilities for the psychoanalyst: questioning clinical experience which cannot reveal anything unless asked precise questions; resorting to history in order to understand the objectification process rather than its result; considering the metapsychological basis of a process whose modalities have formerly been determined. This is what we have tried to do throughout the following pages, our subject being to say, as completely as possible, how to think hypochondria.

Part I
Questions and Problems

Introduction

Abstract The issue of the body invites us to question the Freudian theoretical model. We show why this criticism is required for the study of hypochondria.

For two decades, "return of the body" and "return to the body" have been a convergent focus for many psychiatric and psychoanalytic works; the research and publications that followed vacillated between apology and depreciation, i.e., two opposite forms of fetishization. However, one cannot but notice that this "conversion" strangely resembles a diversion.

Simply put: we lack a theory of the body. Too famous and too fashionable today, the body is indeed an impasse for thought. Established and obvious, ideological and totalitarian, with no possible capacity not to be a thought, this figure has joined the rank of the "obligatory" topics which build up the depressive obsession of a culture and keep thought away from the discovery of its centers. It is generally used with a vague and extremely diffuse meaning, which clearly evidences a theoretical deficiency. Moreover, "body" is not a clearly defined and well-bounded Freudian concept.

But, as the body has no theoretical status in a system which is exclusively conceived in terms of psychical apparatus, the main difficulty is the continuing use of the never questioned Freudian somatization model which opposes and unites the concepts of actual and neurotic. It is also that the compelling questions generated by the body invariably lead to the paradigmatic use of hysteria: as a model, it enables the extension of the conversion process to the pregenital (Sperling 1978); as a norm, it enables multiple conceptions of somatization, all expressed in terms of deprivation (Marty 1980; McDougall 1992). The problem is finally the resulting marginalization of a whole clinical field, both theoretical and practical, considered as a fringe for it is linked to the concept of actual; psychosomatics, psychomotor therapy, psychosis therapy all seem nonintegrable. Paradox of a thought which simultaneously thinks soma as a sort of propping system and as a negative concept.

Founding and constituent on the one hand, marginal and on the fringe on the other hand, burrowed and covered then, the question of the body in psychoanalysis is far from reduced to an internal problem that we would have to examine only from inside, as an integral part of a fully perfected system; therefore, it also constitutes the necessary confrontation which will help re-thinking a problematics. This is a multiple issue: obsolescence and lack of coherence of the definition of soma both considered as a center and an outside; impossibility to use hysteria as a model as it, far from being a pure neurosis, regularly extends beyond the conversional level (Sami-Ali 1987, pp.32–61); frequent coexistence, clinically observed, of multiple bodily symptoms on several levels. Extreme fragility of a conceptual framework.

The only reference framework which clearly integrates hypochondria today seems to be psychoanalysis, but it has to be re-examined and this cannot be done without radically questioning the Freudian somatization model. What are its guiding postulates? What does it objectivize? Thus, if we avoid getting locked in a ready-made system, a new problematics can emerge, free from the prejudice of dichotomy, that will enable us to think both psyche and soma.

Chapter 1
Questions

Abstract Preliminary reflections on the study of hypochondria. We explain that, adjective more than substantive, hypochondria covers a wide nosographic and etiologic spectrum and remains a theoretical blind spot, and also why, more than an entity, it is a problem that questions the contradictions of Freud's theory and the weaknesses of its somatization model. Consequently, the issue of hypochondria induces the need for rigorous and innovative conceptual research. We outline the main features of the comprehensive, critical, and fertile approach that must be defined to create new concepts that extend the frontiers of psychoanalysis and overcome its contradictions while remaining consistent with it. This results in the formulation of our initial questions.

Questions, internal as well as external, so that clinical practice can be interrogated without being imprisoned in a theoretical option. Instead of continuing the previous purely Freudian approach, they must confront all problematics, all contradictions, all theoretical gaps. Negative process, counter-inductive effort. Circle-breaking work whose lineaments can be discovered in literature, in the confrontation of data and problems. Locating the remaining blind spots.

Patchwork of ideas, more often descriptive than explicative, multicolored patchy Harlequin's costume, mixing reflections on actual neuroses to developments on narcissism, the varied readings of hypochondria cannot but strike with their color mismatch and sewing weaknesses.... When we list and question them, we can identify the three research axes that we will have to problematize:

- Adjective rather than substantive,
- Problem rather than entity,
- Negative representation rather than positive content, hypochondria remains quite unexplored.

M. Derzelle, *Towards a Psychosomatic Conception of Hypochondria*,
DOI: 10.1007/978-3-319-03053-1_1,
© Springer International Publishing Switzerland 2014

1.1 Adjective Rather than Substantive

Introductory observation: hypochondria is obviously an indisputable clinical reality, always inseparable from the medical context; however, it seems questionable but also unlikely to find a single and univocal place for it in nosography. It is not a definite entity which can really be diagnosed as such. At the very most, it is a sort of assembly which tends to bring together various clinical pictures, only from a descriptive but never etiological point of view, which all bring out the same concern for the body experienced as ill.

Hidden depression, dejection, and melancholia: since Hippocrates, medical experience, for the specialist as well as for the general practitioner, constantly meets the hypochondriac. This meeting generally results in a shared dissatisfaction between helpless doctors and complaining patients. This constellation of negative affects which endlessly repeats the same sequence is a guiding principle, tenuous but major. For, from extreme confidence—"I've heard of you, you're the only one who can help me"—the suspicious patient switches to defiance—"do you think your treatment will help?"—and then completely nullifies his faith in the next interview—"I feel worse than before." Then exasperation and bad moods will eventually be exchanged as a prelude to rejection, toward a possible elsewhere. Hypochondria as a "climate," at the crossroads of impairment and otherness. But, beyond these shallow responses, what *is* hypochondria?

Between a phenomenological definition and a more semeiological approach, literature is rich but hesitating and leaves the problem unsolved. Symptom pathology? Relational pathology? The first perspective which is the most usual and remains consistent with the classical medical tradition objectivizes signs which pertain to a self-contained system: overstated concern for physical condition, subjectivity of a complaint lacking the weight of the somatic, interpretation of impairment as a simplistic threatening process, withdrawal of concern for the outside world, internal tension and experience of catastrophe. Internally focused on his painful body, the character described as hypochondriacal, locked in and existing as such is, above all, alert to the messages of his coenaestheses even to the most contingent ones. And he interprets them in a negative way. Step by step, opposed to this first intrapsychic approach, the second perspective is inter-psychic. Here, no definition is acceptable unless it implies an interlocutor who, being mute, eloquent, or psittacistic, is nevertheless the one who takes part in the drama. Obligatory partner of his doctor in an inseparable and extremely tragic couple, the character described as hypochondriacal is above all relational (Maurel 1973).

Strange relationship to oneself and/or to another person? This bipolarity can curiously be found on other levels and it seems to insistently underline how hypochondria is linked to ambiguity and even to duality. Double causality, biological or mental, major or minor, delusional or simplex, has always remained out of the reach of any unitary, either nosographic or etiopathogenic, approach. Dual rooting, between body and language: it still remains an object of debate and controversy, located between organogenesis and psychogenesis, genuine illness and mere thematic issue, established delusion and coenaesthesiopathy. Beyond understanding and classification. Alternately neurosis or psychosis. It is no wonder therefore that hypochondria can be found at varying degrees in the whole psychopathological field so that it seems to be its core, but also sunken in it as sheer entity. Center and periphery.

Nevertheless in all cases, whether it is rejected as single entity (Greenfield and Roessler 1958) or considered as an iatrogenic disease of medicalized cultures (Kenyon 1976), it exemplifies the possible links between soma and psyche and cannot be disjointed from a relationship to the world that uses the body as an apparent support medium (Ey 1950). There is then a first question: being an affect-conveying configuration, is hypochondria an unsatisfied demand or a possible genuine label?

This question has no direct and univocal answer. It would imply the possibility of isolating a single underlying process or, at least, of inducing a precise unifying conception. Yet literature shows that this major requisite cannot be met. This is evidenced by Kenyon in a very good 1966 article (Kenyon 1966), where he listed 18 possible usages of the word "hypochondria." Therefore, a purely nosographic conception is invalidated.

> Synonymous with mad or senseless; a mental disease due to a disorder of the digestive tract; term of abuse, i.e., either actually malingering…; general sense of preoccupation with bodily or mental health or functions; personality trait or attribute; a mechanism of defense; neurotic manifestation, especially in lower social classes or in those of poor endowment; an anxiety substitute or affective equivalent; an actual neurosis; closely allied to or a manifestation of neurasthenia or depersonalization; the same as hysteria, only in the male; transitional state between hysteria and psychosis; a nosological entity, primary or essential hypochondriasis; a symptom of almost any of the other commonly recognized psychiatric syndromes, especially depression; prodromal stage of another illness, e.g., schizophrenia; a form of schizophrenia; a form of coenaesthesiopathy; part of a symptomatic psychosis or exogenous reaction.

To which we should add the functional or psychofunctional disorders, as well as dysautonomia, and even the so-called psychosomatic disorders.

As hypochondria is polysemic, it is impossible to *a priori* endow it with a nosological specificity as such, this impossibility being especially reinforced since the medical discourse is increasingly important in our society. Anyway, historically, this recourse to the doctor has replaced the recourse to the priest; unsurprising replacement, as Freud put it as he thought this change was only the abandonment of a so-called "demonological" garment and the taking of another one which was a mere disguise. In this perspective, after Kenyon, we can say that the overflowing extension of the word "hypochondria" undoubtedly justifies that it is no longer really used as a noun but only as an adjective which has a descriptive use. A careful literature review clearly exemplifies this proposal: we have noted down 27 common usages for the adjective "hypochondriacal;" they can be distributed around three major lines: semeiological (neurosis, psychosis, character, delusion, constitution, syndrome, symptom), phenomenological (presentation, recourse, form, idea, concern, theme, worry, grievance, complaint, component, dimension, episode, event, disorder, trend, state, phenomenon, complex), or even ontological (work, drama). Being an adjective more than a substantive, hypo-chondria is a cross-cutting notion. All the attempts to reduce it to a symptom regularly confronted the nosographic obviousness of their senselessness: that is why hypochondria keeps wandering as a stranger who has his seat at the tables of hysteria, depression, psychosis, and actual neurosis.

If hypochondria, clinical picture referring to several diseases, cannot be iden-tified as a medical entity and as it lacks etiological unity, could it find its unity on an exclusively descriptive level? Isn't it, for example, an unsatisfied demand, present in various contexts? Indeed, a real specificity could be found in the complaint itself, in its wording and in the ambivalence of a demand for care whose unifying characteristic is that it is refused, more than in any attempt to give it an etiopathogenic or a nosological definition. Freud did not go into details about this articulation but he nevertheless found two axes in the hypochondriac's very peculiar relationship to the other person: a reversed guiltiness on the one hand (objectal libido), a projected attack against oneself as well as against the other (narcissistic libido), on the other hand. Impossible destruction, impossible healing. Complaint is definitely the element to consider, that is what all authors mean when they persist in situating it in its structural analogy with other relational pathologies: melancholia–mania couple (Fedida 1971; 1975; Ferenczi 1955; Freud 1915[1917]b; Klein 1935; 1940; Araham K), paranoia (Tausk 1933; Abraham K; Klein M), obsessional neurosis (S. Freud). In spite of the variety of the clinical contexts, discourses converge.

As a result of this striking contrast, classification is difficult, that is why opinions diverge. Some authors assume that hypochondria is psychotic (Maurel 1973). Some others consider that no one is totally exempt from this kind of concern (Ey 1950). Some mention it as an irreversible neurosis or last barrier against psychosis. Finally, other authors, more cautious, affirm that theme cannot not prefigure structure. This difficulty is probably the consequence of the notable fact that the hypochondriac's usual discourse is indeed a subversion of medical discourse. The confusion between the medical discourse on hypochondriacs and their own has frequently been noticed (Cottraux 1976). Does the unity of the hypochondriac's discourse lead to a *mise en abyme* in which the doctor sometimes imagines a unity he can call nosological whereas the constant and essential unity is the one he provides without really knowing? The word "observation," ordinarily medical, would not have a one-way meaning here. Discourse unity? Unity of a reduplicated partner? In both cases, the approach remains descriptive. In view of this highly insufficient perspective, let us also find if psychoanalysis can propose an explicative theory for the origin of the disorder of the patient who complains that his body is affected.

On this specific point we must acknowledge our ignorance. When we compare descriptive and explicative levels, we can notice a major discrepancy: super-abundance of descriptions and lack of explanation show how difficult it is to establish a clear theoretical status for the hypochondriacal subject. The main contribution of the psychoanalytical theory is a polymorphous set of scattered words and notions which orderlessly evoke, Oedipus, castration, guiltiness, sadomasochism, anality too, fragmentation sometimes, narcissism mainly, and orality at last. Moreover, this kaleidoscope often sounds like, sometimes straightforwardly, the very hypochondria that it tries to explain. But psychoanalysis remains nebulous on the very strict problem of pathogenesis, quite often referred to with tautologies: "somatic complacency of the organs" (S. Freud), "organ-specific libidinal tonus" (V. Tausk), "yet unknown physiological factor" (O. Fenichel). We must first acknowledge Freud's double contribution. We can sum up Freud's view on hypochondria in the following terms: energetic, economic, cumulative, and quantifying. As for the organ said to be painful, he summons the notion of erogeneity and explains the painful part of the body is libidinally invested and experienced as a penis.

The psychoanalytical theory, either Freud's or his successors,' gives first and foremost a comprehension of the content of fantasy. But as the hypochondriac has a singular way of experiencing his body, his fantasies appear in a singular mode and this might lead us to consider as revocable the Freudian conviction which refuses any sort of "psychical" "signification" (Freud 1916–1917, p.387) to the Actual. Hypochondria is therefore a problem. More than a purely pathogenic explanation, the psychoanalytical theory exposes another version of the text to decipher, text that the hypochondriac tries his best to proclaim, it exposes an explanation that vaguely understands the hypochondriac's experience. Hysterization by psychoanalysis of any pathology outside its scope? Could psychoanalysis be insufficient to grasp the shape and modifications of fantasies even if it is able to describe their content? For instance, the main idea is that, for many hypochondriacs, especially for the ones whose diseased area is in the abdomen or sometimes in the thorax, important pregnancy fantasies are involved. But this position seems incompatible with the Freudian considerations on the penis as prototype of the diseased organ. Unless you produce an amalgam as F. Perrier does when he refers to a "self pregnantified phallus-child." (Perrier 1978, p.241) Interesting but not very clarifying point of view! Anna Freud's point of view was perhaps more significant as she suggested to consider the hypochondriac as an ill child trying to influence his mother through his symptoms and his illness (Freud 1957). Objective description of a nosophobia? Cautious acknowledgement of purely subjective pain sensations? Search for explanation, for signification, for a strange and very paradoxical relationship between two partners? The question remains.

1.2 Problem Rather than Entity

Second obvious fact: cross-cutting designation with multiple uses, alternately pathogenic or iatrogenic, sociogenic too, hypochondria remains undoubtedly problematic on a strict theoretical level. It provides more questions than answers or solutions. At the very most, it is a sort of complex which questions the essential principles of thought in its formal logic: ubiquity, ambiguity, and contradiction require us to take into account its complexity and to dismiss dogmas and conformity as well.

First of all, ubiquity, at least under three forms. The first one, expressed in literature with various terms as articulation, "pre-psychotic" period or "actual core," gives hypochondria a pivotal position. In his works Freud exemplifies this position several times, following his usual evolutionist approach that goes from simplest to most complex. For instance, he added a footnote to his text about president Schreber:

> I shall not consider any theory of paranoia trustworthy unless it also covers the hypo-chondriacal symptoms by which this disorder is almost invariably accompanied. It seems to me that hypochondria stands in the same relation to paranoia as anxiety neurosis does to hysteria (Freud 1911, p.303, note 2)

and he added, in 1914:

> I have said before that I am inclined to class hypochondria with neurasthenia and anxiety neurosis as a third "actual" neurosis. It would probably not be going too far to suppose that in the case of the other neuroses a small amount of hypochondria was regularly formed at the same time (Freud 1914, p.83).

Much more than a state, hypochondria is here a reference-term referring to the concept of relationship: it is as if its study created a sort of family like structure between all pathologies. Can it possibly be considered as the moment when the patient enters into an illness? It is true if we listen to all the words which depict it as the modification of a *status quo ante*, dimension of a change whose dramatic experience Freud underlined in the Schreber case: the libido withdrawal from the outside world gets the proportion of an "internal catastrophe" which can only be subsumed by the idea of end of the world.

The second one, referring to a definition which favors the "symptom pathology" aspect, i.e., the aspect of a syndrome affecting a self-contained system, gives hypochondria a unique position: being co-extensive to any pathology. Like body image, it seems to be in all the places where something is missing in one of the processes that should result in the creation either of a specific identity (I am somebody) or of a sexed identification (I am somebody, a man or a woman). Thus we can see the hypochondriacal shadow hang around whenever a psychical or somatic symptom cuts into body image integrity. The hysteric, endlessly questioning his sexed self (who am I, a man or a woman?) cannot but expose polymorphous pains which inhibit both his life and sexuality. The obsessive patient, questioning his own existence (am I dead or alive?) and for whom the fact of "feeling" represents a danger, will prefer to think his deep anxiety through a precise and minute study of all the sensations he comes to feel. The depressed one then, on whom the "shadow of object," of the so much loved lost object, has fallen down, will perceive the inside of his body as bad, putrefied, sometimes dead or at least absent. The schizophrenic one will see strangeness everywhere when it comes to his body, totally or partly possessed by another and experienced as elsewhere. As for the paranoid, if he suffers in his body, it is because a persecutor keeps altering it with a ceaseless ingenuity. All those pathological cases only reproduce, in their caricatures, an alleged health called normality. Because who can escape this kind of concern on body condition, on corporeity?

The third one, which is food for thought on the difficulty to draw limits between a "normal complex," known as hypochondriacal (Ey 1950, p.453) which would be immanent in human nature, and extreme frankly pathological forms, sees hypochondria as a sort of continuum whose reality would be the one of a psychopathological structure of human life. Whenever a perception, or even a simple idea, concerning our body, is interpreted as having the value of a definite lesion, it is a specifically hypochondriacal "theme." For example, when we feel a commonplace pain, we all happen to vaguely imagine either a heart or brain impairment, or a poisoning caused by constipation. Hypochondria tells the mystery of the body whose fragility grips our "entrails." All that concerns viscera, organic functions, medical acts and fear of death consequently creates a great unrest within all of us, as the deep echo of "primary narcissism." We must consequently be aware that it is the backdrop, primary self-consciousness as somatic matter, condition and partner of all reality which heavily influences our psychical life, and constantly attracts it toward somatic anxiety by creating catastrophe images. That is why, undoubtedly, hypochondria fundamentally links up with the difficult problem of anxiety and might only be one of its aspects. Structure of existence turned into a form of existence?

Ambiguity then, whose essential mode can be found in a debate that began in the eighteenth century and questions the legitimacy of a binary distinction between two disorders, depending on whether its form is "major" or "minor." Two centuries later, this debate can be summed up this way on the nosographic level: should we define two forms of hypochondria, a "simple" or "neurotic" one for "conscious" patients, and a "delusional," "psychotic," or "vesanic" one, or should we admit the unity of this symptom? This question, which is still pending in the twentieth century (Codet 1939), alternately received two answers, depending on whether it was considered on the theoretical level or corresponded to a natural clinical division on the nosographic level. Criteria greatly vary here. For Esquirol, thus, some patients must be put aside, the ones who

> are deluding themselves on the intensity of their suffering, but... do not lose their mind unless lypomania complicates hypochondria.

Foville supports the same distinction:

> he does not want, Cotard writes, lucid hypochondriacs to be confused with insane hypochondriacs, hypochondria itself with hypochondriacal delusion.

Under the condition, however, that insanity, a purely social criterion, could be a sufficient argument:

> People with a persecutory delusion, not intense, with a light degree of mental depression... and with so many other mental disorders that are only identified by the doctor, are in the same case as hypochondria! For us, there is no nosological difference: hypochondria is a prelude, an attenuate form, but it is vesanic as well as hypochondriacal delusion in confirmed madness (Cotard 1891).

Vigorous profession of hypochondria as one, on the background of an eternal dual polarity.

Even if its unicity, always oriented toward psychosis, is clearly stated by Freud, by Cotard, by Pinel or by Ey, these authors, at the same time, produce an ambiguous discourse charged with duality. Henri Ey, for instance, chooses the singular in the title of his famous study n. 17: "Hypochondria." He nevertheless distinguishes two major clinical pictures, classically split into two hypochondriae, a "minor" one and a delusional one, depending on the structure into which they fit. In the various presentations of the same hypochondriacal phenomenon, in spite of levels and disparities linked to "background" and "personal characteristics," it seems that a delusional theme, whether of jealousy, grandeur, or influence, constitutes a way of situating oneself in the world that, to some degree, has a form of homogeneity. Of speech, of listening, of relation to the other person. Same bipolarity in Freud's works. If no allusion to a scission between two possible forms of hypochondria can be found in any of them, if always and everywhere he calls it neurosis—a word we often understand as psychosis as, until 1924 approximately, "narcissistic neuroses" were chronic psychoses—in short, if it is the core of paraphrenia, his multiple notations nevertheless burdened the following research with a major double pitfall: the one of considering hypochondria as an actual disorder, purely somatic, which will turn it into an "actual neurosis," an actual organ neurosis, and the one of considering it as a regression to primary narcissism, a libidinal withdrawal on a pure organ-ego which will classify it among psychoses.

Admittedly, it is difficult to apprehend hypochondria as an actual neurosis as well as a disorder defined as narcissistic and Freud never attempted to provide a more coherent theorization. It is perhaps the therapeutic point of view that determined him toward actuality as, like his successors, he quickly noticed that analysis was unproductive. Besides, Freud as an analyst had a famous failure with the "Wolf Man" who, several years after his analysis, evolved toward a frank and well-defined psychosis whose theme was precisely very hypochondriacal. But we must notice that this ambiguity, never solved and always continued, is the starting point of some interpretations which look like a compromise. Fenichel's thesis exemplifies it by building a borderline concept between actual neurosis and chronic psychosis (!):

> Hypochondriasis is an organ neurosis whose physiological factor is still unknown; it may
> be brought about by a primary hypocathexis of the organ representations (in psychoses), or
> by primary unknown organic manifestations of the state of being dammed up (in actual
> neuroses) (Fenichel 1946).

From this investment of a representation to a body image disturbance (Schilder 1935), hypochondria might be turned into hysteric neurosis by the pregnant allusion to a fantasy system. Even if we admit that it always refers to the first stages of the ego in its bodily form, such a hypochondria is not actual at all, whereas Freud always maintained this quality, that is precisely a lack of fantasy.

Contradiction, at last, linked to the "status" of hypochondria in the Freudian system, both reflects and results from the very conception of a register of the actual, being itself connected with a theory that, with the aim of considering and elaborating the important question of somatizations, presents a two-dimension model using, above all, the opposition between psychoneurotic and actual as a model. Pertinently qualified as bi-dimensional by M. Sami-Ali (Sami-Ali 1982), this last model consists in admitting that, opposed to the psychoneurotic symptoms which always refer to the repressed, to repression failure, possibly through a somatic expression, actual neurosis (hypochondria, anxiety neurosis, neurasthenia) symptoms result, with no mediation, from possible disturbances of the sexual metabolism whose decrease or increase they reveal, with no meaning. They are, as Freud says when he evokes them as:

> intracranial pressure, sensations of pain, a state of irritation in an organ, weakening or inhibition of a function (Freud 1916–1917, p.387)

meaningless symptoms. Opposed to the primary meaning of psychoneurotic symptoms, they can only have a secondary one, acquired afterwards, that does not trigger the symptom formation process, which keeps them fundamentally apart from all etiological symbol system. Consequently, actual symptoms are, for Freud, purely physical.

> They are not only manifested in the body (as are hysterical symptoms, for instance, as well), but they are also themselves entirely somatic processes, in the generating of which all the complicated mental mechanisms we have come to know are absent (Freud 1916–1917, p.387).

But let us have a look at the critical moment when, unveiling the complications, we ask how actual and neurotic articulate. Freud finds the missing link in his evolutionist conception: actual precedes neurotic as minerals precede granitic rocks, according to a transformation rule where elements gradually complexify. There is thus

> between the symptoms of actual neuroses and the ones of psychoneuroses, an interesting relation that greatly contributes to the knowledge of the symptomatic formation of the latter: the symptom of actual neurosis is often the core and the preliminary phase of the psychoneurotic one (Freud 1916–1917, p.390).

This elegant and interesting phrase has a mainly theoretical orientation which obviously shows that this conception results from some problems with nosography and perhaps pathogeny, but which, against reason, contains a hidden and unlikely contradiction. If sexuality is, in actual neuroses, genital and adult-specific, it is on the contrary pregenital and child-specific in neurotic disorders. Considering that actual states precede neurotic states is an inversion of chronology, the adult being in a strange position before the child! Freud did not ignore that this contradiction inhered in his conception that is why he called it a "disgraceful lacuna" (Jones 1955, pp.502–503) in his theory and he acknowledged that nothing "coherent" emerged from his ideas. However he maintained this distinction, this dichotomy, throughout his reflections, and bequeathed the resulting aporia, first and complete, to us.

Of course, it is the same when Freud presents hypochondria as a preparation to paranoia, as the elaboration of an actual anxiety (therefore genital) fixed to the body, coupled with the belief that this always happens according to a linear process by gradual complexification. But is hypochondria really simpler than paranoia?

Nothing is less certain. Nothing ensures that etiology could be reduced to the purely actual processes. This is exemplified by the numerous nuances used by Freud's exegetes: to avoid seeing or pointing this contradiction, they neutralize it with an oft-repeated *petitio principii* which is that actual is the background of neurotic. In this respect, Nunberg is a good example when he mentions the case of a man who, having used coitus interruptus for a long time, suffers from a great anxiety of bodily nature.

> The patient felt throughout his body what another man feels in his genitalia when he is sexually aroused. He identified his whole body with his genitalia.... The fear of losing parts of his body unconsciously corresponded to the fear of losing his genitalia; it was therefore a castration anxiety. As a result of the disruption of the discharge of sexual products in coitus, there was apparently a libido accumulation that extended to the body.... The ego was defending against the resulting feelings of pain, with the help of the former unconscious castration anxiety, which was then expressed in the hypochondriacal sensations and fears (Nunberg 1932).

In this example, anxiety explains the use of coitus interruptus, presumed cause of hypochondria, and not the other way round: in the logic of the Freudian system, this contradiction is unavoidable.

1.3 Negative Representation Rather than Positive Content

Last obvious fact: double-sense question, terrible, and sweet torment that patient and doctor administrate each other in vain, hypochondria has the characteristic of holding the discourse of its diagnosers. It resembles an echo of the medical language finally concluding that "this patient is not ill." Strange designation whose negative form can also be found in the psychoanalytic approach to maintain Actual as a negativity, as if the Medical constituted its backing. Does hypochondria tells an ideology whose relay would be negative thought?

The key of the debate concerning the concept of actual resides, on this precise point, in the central notion of normativity whose two complementary modalities tell all its influence on the Freudian model. Paradigmatic utilization of hysteria to which invariably lead any questioning proceeding from the body, consequent marginalization of an entire clinical field, considered on the fringe for linked to the Actual. Negativity, thus, of actual neurosis on the background of the positivity of psychoneurosis, which is constantly regarded as the norm even when one diverts from it, and even deliberately. It is consequently no wonder then to see the theories known as psychosomatic, no matter when they appeared, from S. Ferenczi's "organ neurosis" to P. Marty's "psychosomatic order," ordinarily referring to the actual, remain closely linked to neurosis and particularly to hysteria. Permanently, and throughout history, with links liable to be dually defined: positively first, the latter having a model status for the former (Alexander 1965; Dunbar), but also negatively, with an effort to show the existence of symptoms which can be called deficient, which would predispose to somatizations, where psychoneurosis is taken as exclusive norm even if "it consists in missing mechanisms with no extra mechanisms" (Marty 1980). Negative expressions, faltering ego, general negativity of signs, vanishing of mental elaboration, follow one another to produce a "debossed" picture, fundamentally situated using deprivation, and even deficit, relationship to the organization known as psychoneurotic. Hypochondria as actual neurosis is in good part a reality created by what we can call this system of thought.

To this is added a preferential link, soon outlined by Freud (1895) between aging and actual neuroses, both thought as theoretical evidences of a biological order seen as failing, and which would be two forms of "weakening." Based on a quantitative pathogeny which Freud would maintain in 1937, this explicit relationship between senescence and anxiety neurosis—this anxiety, taking another direction, and deflecting inwards, results in hypochondria—definitely establishes a strict analogy that is of status:

> There are men who, as women, reach a critical age and develop an anxiety neurosis at the time when their potency decreases and libido increases (Freud 1894, p.26).

No possible doubt on this disorder's origin: it is an increase of sexual arousal only resulting from biological processes, which cannot decrease either because of a "relative psychical insufficiency" to master it or release it, or because the outside world presently opposes its possible and real outflow whereas it "could have given satisfaction to a smaller demand." Neurosis or psychosis, intra- or extra- subjective, the disturbance remains quantitative. It is a dysfunction or an insufficiency. As a consequence we can say that this negativity characterizes hypochondria, all the more because the "arganic" complaint is very frequent and manifest during aging. Psychoneurosis used as a reference would correspond to a positivity probably represented by a young adult man, a child, an egg maybe! In short by social or cultural ideals based on the notion of productivity. Idealization of an anteriority which dooms time, thought as linearized, to be of no return and destructive.

In this respect, it is important to notice that, as aging, hypochondria only seems apt to be seen as an involution. Hypochondria's meaningful aspects as an impairment constantly expressed by questioning the meaning of pure quantity, of lack and absence of any kind of psychical object, echo the purely negative ones of aging which are constantly expressed as "loss," "decline," "destruction" or "weakness." Whether their "causes" are searched for in the outside world, in the subject or in the production of a notably increased actual libido, everything seems to happen as if the source of fantasy had dried up, producing a psychical void into which the reality of body and "socius" are at the same time engulfed. For the pathogeny invoked in the actual phenomena, as sexual abstinence or coitus interruptus, which is above all an absence of release, is also a failure of the relation to the other person, impossible meeting and lack of pleasure. As a consequence, the strictly medical perspective yields the project of healing, at least ideally, through active, actual and immediate correction of the triggering factor, in the real world.

It follows from what I have said that neuroses are entirely preventible as well as incurable. The physician's task is wholly shifted on to prophylaxis (Freud 1887–1904, p.184).

or

In such a case, the doctor naturally applies an actual therapy using the modification of sexual physical activity and he is right to do so if his diagnosis is correct (Freud 1887–1904, p.184).

This reveals the well-known typical medical attitude which tends to use therapy to confirm a diagnosis whose basis is a semiology-based etiology. This also reveals that actual neuroses can only be maintained and defined by Freud through the surprising use of the negative in a non-analytical approach. For when they are propping on a semiology which vanishes under the effect of reality, they ask an important question: has a foreign founding model been imported into psychoanalysis? Hypochondria: medical prototype of a lack?

The Negative indeed seems consubstantial to it. From a general point of view there is, for actual neuroses, no real definition, acceptable as distinct and "in itself," except on the clinical level: they are either defined by reference to the Psychoneurotic, triumph of negative thought, or to the Medical, triumph of normative thought. In both cases, the hypochondriac adds the special feature of being known as "impossible to treat." Object of almost inexhaustible questionings as the body which only suffers in its complaint, free from damage or dysfunction, constitutes a real enigma, it perfectly embodies the total escape from medical power. The hypochondriac's symptoms are purely somatic, in their pathogeny and their clinical expression, symptoms which are meaningless, sometimes even expressed in a senseless form, hypochondria is no indication for analysis and seems to remain opaque to investigation, and as anxiety neurosis patients, hypochondriacs, Lebovici writes

develop no clear neurotic symptoms and experience reality as the object of direct suffering, without constructing fantasies.... Deficiency of narcissistic organization makes them able of partial and transitional, objectal investments; this makes psychoanalytic cure virtually impossible, and justifies the term proposed by P. Marty, of behavior neurosis (Lebovici 1969).

Resigned and powerless or listening but annoyed: the doctor as well as the analyst are questioned by the hypochondriac's performance.

As analytical listening is impossible for actual neurosis, we have to focus on the objectification process which produced it. Just as aging and anxiety neurosis have had the same sort of pathogeny since the early times of psychoanalysis, it is interesting to point out that the forbidden listening, from a technical point of view, was stated by Freud ten years later (1904–1905), when Freud exposed that the age of fifty, which was nearly his own at that time, was a counter-indication, establishing again a link between the concept of actual and senescence:

If the patient is in the neighborhood of the fifties, the conditions for psycho-analysis become unfavorable, because the bulk of psychic material can no more be studied thoroughly, the cure is too prolonged, and the capacity to make psychic processes go backwards is weakening (Freud 1904[1903], p.254).

what he will later call "lack of plasticity of the psychical process" reminds of the "rigidity," the "resistance to change" which is frequently said to characterize the elderly: "old people are no more educable." Listening to the elderly is then forbidden in three ways, which are in the end applicable to the hypochondriac. Theoretical impossibility, due to an economic pathogeny which is purely somatic and thus comparable to the impossible listening of actual neuroses and their insufficient mentalization: i.e., failure to hear the body. Technical impossibility due to an excessive mass of psychical material and to an important resistance to change: i.e., failure to hear Actuality. Impossibility, finally, of any listening in crisis situation which is not uncommon,

> The ego's whole interest is taken by the painful reality and it withholds itself from analysis (Freud 1937, p.232)

i.e., failure to hear the Real. Three proscriptions which are hardly supported by clinical experience and finally result in classifying those counter-indications along a total *a priori* denial.

They ask many questions as they reduce the cause to its effect whose meaning could be de-signified by an analyst's ear. Is the extreme difficulty to adapt listening necessarily an impossibility? What is hidden behind this "rigidity" presented first of all as a difficulty to make the psychical process go backwards, for this "making" could be achieved by the subject as well as by his psychoanalyst? Finally, has the mentalization insufficiency with disturbance of the somatic order, always considered as the biological order, no meaning which would simply exclude a linguistic version of the actual phenomena? Hypochondria shows that the subject of the debate, concerning norm, is a "translation that cannot work." It gives no understandable text, neither on the level of a possible therapeutic effect, nor in the technical and theoretical report which could constitute the desired formula. Some authors then claim that those symptoms are not a language, that they "mean nothing." Untenable position, since meaninglessness is enunciated in the register of meaning, otherwise it could not even be formulated. Therefore it has a meaning, which is a meta-meaning that has to be seen and scrutinized. Thus, what we designate as a denial of meaning for psychoanalysis is first the symptom itself, then its subject, and then the psychoanalyst and even psychoanalysis itself! What then can we say but that the meaning of meaninglessness is to be found first toward a fantasy, only on condition that we integrate into it the speaker's and the interlocutor's?

Therefore, a multifaceted aporia emerges from the Freudian model of somatization, produced by a systematizing approach permanently inspired by evolutionism and classifying phenomena in gradually complexifying series. The links between psychical and somatic, for instance, require to be thought in terms that are different from the concepts of Propping and Actual considered as the core of Neurotic. This thought on the body used to be the cornerstone of diverging models, it cannot imagine the action of a process which is as real as imaginary, it is then nothing but a theoretical gap. Positive side of the negative neurotic symptom, actual phenomena then seem to belong to the perverse register. But there is another theoretical gap: hypochondria, linearly thought as "pre-psychotic," i.e., actual core of paranoia, when Freud called it "psychosis," rejecting both psychical and somatic toward the same "hypothetical" purity:

> I shall not consider any theory of paranoia trustworthy unless it also covers the *hypochondriacal* symptoms by which this disorder is almost invariably accompanied (Freud 1911, pp.56–57).

If, for the hypochondriac, there is never any isolated physical symptom at all, if there is always also a delusional thought feeding on various dysmorphophobia, the entire problem must be rethought for it reveals the failure of an evolutive scheme: projection precedes and follows projection. Consequently, this Freudian deficiency is threefold as it first concerns hypochondria, then paranoia and finally projection. Hypochondria must therefore be entirely rethought in its dual relation with projection and somatization: the Schreberian episode known as hypochondriacal is, from this point of view, quite relevant as it is a temporary counterpart of paranoia.

Hypochondria is indeed a delusion of the body due to a projection which prevents the belief in a mysteriously impaired body from ever changing: this simple fact definitely undermines the Freudian somatization model whose finality is to articulate Somatic and Psychical, Actual and Neurotic, in an identical chronological historic precedence. If the Freudian principle of an actual genesis and a simple structure of hypochondria as a prelude to psychosis turns out to be inapplicable, then another model must be elaborated, a model which enables to think a coexistence, far from any linear causal conception. Therefore, this requires the proof of the projective aspect of hypochondria, a requirement which reminds of a problematics whose analysis was promised by Freud, but never realized. The absence of a theoretical status of hypochondria which would enable to think it clearly is then closely linked to the underlying absence of a theoretical status for projection. The Schreber case definitely exemplifies this problem that Freud had to struggle with. On two counts at least. What is projection? On this question there are two very different perspectives which are open to interpretation and which never give a real answer: first, the one of symptomatic formation and then, the one of repression, which has become more classical. In both cases, as a real aporia and a never taken necessary detour, projection stands, and cannot be reduced to its only function known as pathognomonic.

> The thorough examination of the process of projection that we have postponed to another occasion will provide the certitudes that are still missing (Freud 1911; 1912–1913; 1915[1917]a).

Retrospectively, it is this uncertainty that holds together the entire Freudian system.

Lack of a sufficient theory of the body and lack of a clear status of hypochondria thus come very close to form a theoretical conceptual void: one where projection is regularly thought, on the clinical level, as a function, defensive but not elaborated in a global work beyond the psychopathological field, according to Freud's never fulfilled wish. After three decades (1894–1927) of successive milestones, of eclipses followed by sudden resurgences, the mystery of the body is still there, it is the mystery of the subject's relation to his body as well as to the world, and it constantly brings back under the hand of Freud the problem of the link, of the bridge, of the *vinculum* with the concepts of somatic and physiologic. Clinically obvious in all constant well-known and knowable symptoms that are those of anxiety, it greatly resists elucidation, regardless of the theories and names: mysterious jump, actual factor, predisposition, choice of neurosis, distinction between real and neurotic anxiety, trauma, real, anxiety theories. As hypochondria, the concept of anxiety, which bounds an important but difficult field, is often together with a double clinical and statutory requirement which points out, as missing, the theorization of a body synchronically both subject and object: at one end, anxiety is physical, expressed in physical or somatic signs, at the other end it is intrinsically linked to the subject and can be named with the scholastic term of ipseity. That is to say how much hypochondria, anxiety, projection, and body are essentially linked in a problematics which has to be explained.

> If we cannot see things clearly we will at least see clearly what the obscurities are (Freud 1925, 124).

Guided by this motto which used to be Freud's, we are now able to put into words the three questions resulting from our three axes:

- Adjective more than substantive: what distinguishes hypochondria as a problematics?
- Problem more than entity: how can we think a resolution of the contradictions that inhere in it as well as in the concept of actual neurosis?
- Normativity more than reality: What positive content can we give to an entirely negative designation, created by a normative system of thought?

What object to think? With which concepts that would enable to avoid contradiction? to avoid being locked in any sort of system?

Chapter 2
Problems

Abstract We show how the different theoretical obstacles to the conceptualization of hypochondria, its characterization as an actual neurosis, must be questioned, as well as the Actual-Neurotic duality itself. As this dichotomy structures the Freudian system, we explain why its main corollaries must be criticized. Another obstacle must be studied, that is the absence of theoretical status of the body in psychoanalysis. These in-depth analyses lead us to fruitful research perspectives.

The problem is about going beyond. Beyond a conceptual model, which is simple on the theoretical level but reflects the complexity of things as well, a model that however becomes obsolete as soon as it confronts clinical reality which resists simplifications, only offering mixed cases. Beyond a system which turns from hypothesis to system when, instead of being used for empiric data interpretation, it is used in order to create an object projectively, always shaping it in its own image, making it analytically uninterpretable. Beyond a diptych-like framework, possibly likely to be dually read as the overflowing of hypochondria into hysteria, on the organic level as well as on the psychotic level, symmetrically corresponds to the overflowing of hypochondria in the psychotic field as a so-called Actual neurosis (Sami-Ali 1987).

The present work thus constitutes the half of a vast perspective aiming at entirely rethinking concepts: like hypochondria, hysteria raises a problem, as it makes several levels coexist. Two ways are then possible to begin a research between biology and psychoanalysis: their common point is that they break a conformity⋯

2.1 Hindrance to Thinking

The drastic epistemological gap between actual and psychoneurosis, even if it is a framework for thought, is nevertheless a terrible and constant obstacle to thought linked to the indisputable transformation of psychoanalysis into an ideology. For the contradiction which inheres in the system itself, and has no alternative but the vicious circle, shows how much the Freudian project is a projection which articulates onto another one that is the illusion of a "primitivity". Permanent attempt to

M. Derzelle, *Towards a Psychosomatic Conception of Hypochondria*,
DOI: 10.1007/978-3-319-03053-1_2,
© Springer International Publishing Switzerland 2014

make coincide an "inside" which belongs to the imaginary and a real "outside" which seems to conform to it, representing a specific case, the Freudian model is also a temptation to escape reality test by becoming an almost uncontested dogma where all dimensions of thought have disappeared (See Fig. 2.1).

Three characteristics distinguish this system and define, more than a method specific to discovery, a view adapted to exposition, wording, and transmission:

- Form: a dualist thought, more aimed at maintaining internal coherence than at expressing observed facts, reveals a need for systematization.
- Content: the idea of evolution, "fundamental language" common to many nineteenth century authors, enables extrapolation and, analogically, extension of the specific psychoanalytic principles out of the psychoanalytical field.
- Theory: a diachronic model which, as M. Foucault powerfully outlined it, prevailed throughout the West in the nineteenth century (Foucault 1966), insists on the permanent interdependence with what has come before, considered as antecedent.

Hypochondria meets this obstacle to thought which is situated in history and results from history.

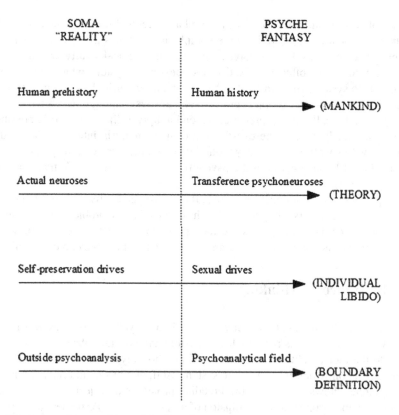

Fig. 2.1 Structural isomorphism of the Freudian system

- Dualism first, under the sterile form of the Actual/Neurotic pair, which shares with many others the grim privilege of giving a globalizing view of human and biological evolution, so that this view seems a projection of multiple clinical observations: Reality/Fantasy, Somatic/Psychical, Self preservation/Sexual. Let us name them "synthetic concepts," by their single aim which seems close to the great explanatory myths which account for the totality of each phenomenon. They contrast with the more clinical, and perhaps analytical, concepts which, as transference, enable discovery and, through experience, remain in direct contact. Dualism is not, therefore, the essential problem. Even if it is an obstacle to research and discovery, it can also be particularly fruitful when it is a purely confrontational notion, basis of how psychical life works, and from which the solutions that are psychoneuroses develop. We should rather isolate two different uses which coexist in the Freudian system and which the different drive theories successively exemplify: if the former, which is anchored to clinical practice, fruitfully produced a model where conflict is predominant and even receives a corporeal foundation while remaining internal to the analytical field, the latter, on the contrary, is terribly sterilizing as it opposes life instincts to death instincts, thus producing a self-contained system which, on the clinical level, has no justification. A synthetic concept blocks all exits, intending to explain all and nothing at the same time: a self-confirming dogma can follow from it which, as an all-embracing vision, tells orthodoxy, focal point of coteries. The concept of actual is akin to this use: one can be for or against it, debate is not possible.
- Evolutionism then, which, via analogy, that is via a reflection whose very purpose is to excuse from scientific work, enables to establish a structural iso-morphism where actual is identified with simple, with inferior, with almost archaic. Projected on the level of world history and helped by a cyclical tem-porality, hypochondria becomes the "primordial primitive," initial stage toward which one comes to regress and to which one sometimes even remains fixed: regression to the narcissistic phase, the one of early childhood which is repro-duction of the narcissistic phase of all humanity. In plain language: the Actual neurotic is a version of the baby and of the caveman too! It is no use to insist on its rejection from the psychoanalytical field··· The "archaic illusion" is thus triumphant, formal similarity hiding the greatest heterogeneity. But, as well as for the uncanny, extrapolation seems to be the rule:

> The double was originally an insurance against the extinction of the self···, and it seems likely that the "immortal" soul was the first double of the body. The invention of such doubling as a defense against annihilation that has a counterpart in the language of dreams, which is fond of expressing the idea of castration by duplicating or multiplying the genital symbol. In the civilization of Ancient Egypt, it became a spur to artists to form images of the dead in durable materials. But these ideas arose on the soil of boundless self-love, the primordial narcissism that dominates the mental life of both the child and primitive man and when this phase is surmounted, the meaning of the "double" changes: having been once an insurance of immortality, it becomes the uncanny harbinger of death (Freud 1919).

Infantile is equated with anteriority.

- Diachrony, finally, which is going beyond and preserving an "Actual" core in any psychoneurosis, thus defining a genealogy where evolutionism is unifying: in addition to the fact that simple precedes complex which is always propped on an inferior form, this method always isolates a causal chain which explains superior forms by elementary factors. Such a thought is thus hierarchic, as it goes from Somatic to Psychological posing Actual precedes Psychoneurotic; it conforms to Spencerian evolutionism which is only a sociobiological by-product of Darwinism deviated toward liberalism by the argument, shaped as a simulacrum, of a naturally highly nonegalitarian order (Tort 1983, pp.333–431). As a consequence, the diachronic model which asserts that either paranoia or paraphrenia derive, through a strict causality, from hypochondria, considered as little elaborated, is just a form of the ideology that prevailed in the early eighteenth century, in its attempt to define a genuinely scientific framework. The classical scientific Cartesian method which links the facts to be explained to their causes is then an alibi for an ideology that can be called para-scientific.

Hypochondria is thus an impeded thought as long as it remains imprisoned in a conceptual framework whose conformity to an external model seems to have been Freud's and his successors' main concern, even at a very high cost: absolute privilege of an internal coherence over the total comprehension of clinical experience, possible exclusion of a part of it rather than rejection of the founding illusion. Hence an improper structural isomorphism can be found even in the paradox: even if he continually tried to expel them from the strict limits of psychoanalysis, Freud always wanted to keep actual neuroses all the way in all their complexity.

> I had no more opportunity later to return to the investigation of Actual neuroses. This part of my work has not either been taken over by others. Today when I consider the results I had achieved then, I have to recognize that they were as a primitive and schematic representation of a State of things that was probably more complex. But they basically still seem fair good today. I would have gladly subsequently submitted to a psychoanalytic review other cases of pure juvenile neurasthenia; this could unfortunately not be done. To give indications on some incorrect interpretations, I want to emphasize here that I am far from denying the existence of psychic conflicts and neurotic complexes in neurasthenia. I only maintain that these patients' symptoms are neither mentally determined nor analytically resoluble, but should be thought of as the direct toxic consequences of the disturbed sexual chemism (Freud 1984, pp.44–45).

Was this a sign of Freud's desire, comparable to Schlieman's, to legitimize in the realities he dug up, in any elaboration or proof that he could point out as a reality? There would only be then, for hypochondria as actual neurosis a theoretical interest: the one of propping the Psychoneurotic, enabling us then, through negative logic, to define what is legitimately analytic.

2.2 The Dimension of Thought

Reintroducing the dimension of thought where there is in fact only a commonplace reflection, shaped by conformity and conform to a "ready-thought" posited as truth, this necessity becomes obvious for whom has noticed how the Freudian model results in impasses. A double obstacle must especially be addressed: the one of the contradiction specific to the concept of actual, and the one of a total lack of theoretical status for hypochondria, ignored in the *Vocabulaire de la psychanalyse* (Laplanche and Pontalis 1967, p.177), where anxiety neurosis (Laplanche and Pontalis 1967, p.274) and neurasthenia (Laplanche and Pontalis 1967, p.265) find their natural place. We must think to distance ourselves and thus to leave the maternal and primary way of thinking whose gaps we can see.

Rupture? Transgression? Revolt? Projection? Point out the mother's mistake to think something new? Tell oneself and acknowledge that she has proved "passable". As

mothers, masters, passable analysts, are the ones who reveal insufficient from the beginning (Schneider 1982),

in the same sense as, in 1937 (Freud 1937), Freud said that the analyst was bound to be insufficient when he considered the crazy task that he had undertaken. They are the ones who never turn "giving food for thought" into "producing thought."

What is lost, from the first phrase to the second one, is the internalization of a mandatory model with which one feels as one without seeing that it constitutes an impediment to think. Dogma forbids discovery. Then come struggle against many resistances, choice of an approach, compliance with requirements.

1. Resistances, encountered at the time of a first research "pre-text" which proposed to try to sketch an intelligibility model for somatic complaint, based on concrete clinical material—the "negative reports"—and finding a guiding thread in the use of hypochondria, a key focus, much more than a structure or a diagnosis. This use finally led us to two major obstacles, restricting the elaboration of practical experience. The first one consisted in the fact that Actual was posited as desperately defined "off limits": sheer denial from which the analytical game results, which is a double exclusion of reality in its social as well as biological form, and which any discourse on the concept of actual, hence on hypochondria, encounters. The second one concerned the theoretical gap specific to hypochondria which uncannily echoes the "insufficiency" of psychical elaboration, outlined by the Freudian discourse, as if it was the analytical field's. A third obstacle also arose, another gap: the almost nonexistent community rivalry and internal wars on the subject of an elaboration by the analysts themselves who, concerned with exegesis exercises, continually unanimously outlawed actual neuroses. When we survey the analytical field what we see is neither gradation, nor readable fading, but precise, forced, and clear-cut boundary stones.

2. Various paths to tackle this wide-scope problematics, never discussed in want of confrontation with the necessity of multiple off-center shifts. The first one consists in an attempt to tightly elaborate a theoretical reflection, as close as possible to clinical experience to which specific questions are asked and which helps assessing exactly the gap between the concrete collected material and what seems to be an "obligatory way of thinking". It is difficult to do so, not only because of the multiple registers to refer to (somatic depression, thymic disorder field, narcissism, masochism, psychosomatic sphere), but also because of a dual hindrance: the one of an almost total exteriority of this theoretical grafting to the existing corpus, the one of maintaining an uneasy distance from the Freudian as well as from the patients' discourse. The second perspective consists in rather questioning from inside, having noticed a major absence in all the stages of the former path: the one of a general theory of the body where the lack of a specific status of hypochondria seems to be a variation, a specific case. From this point of view, the identified theoretical gap concerns and questions the theoretical and conceptual apparatus of psychoanalysis, inducing the following interrogations: what else must we think? What can we think otherwise that, giving the psychoanalytical thought a relevant somatization model would make it possible to think hypochondria as a clinical reality on the explanatory more than descriptive level? Both paths draw a to and fro cycle between experience and conceptualization: they lead to a clearer view of the former and to a greater theoretical refinement of elaboration.

3. Resistances and routes have a plural form. These remarks thus introduce the necessity, to justify the chosen approach, that the two fundamental requirements ordinarily guiding any theoretical work be met by the conceptualization to discover, presently missing. It first has to produce a theorization apt to account for the known and acknowledged facts explained by the previous theory as well as other still unexplained ones: this is where its criterion of economy lies. Secondly, it has to make it possible to predict new facts that it would help to discover, which means that, in this respect, it must include hypotheses opening on new findings and have thus an anticipatory function: that is where its heuristic criterion lies. Hypochondria seen as an impeded thought. This wording shows how ignorance and lack of explanation characterize this issue: in a given theoretical and historical moment, it reveals the limits of our reflection.

2.3 Thinking Differently

Let us finally add, as regards requirements, that we must take into account the lineaments resulting from the study of literature which points out the murky nature of hypochondria. Indeed, the conceptualization which we are seeking seems gradually definable, through successive approximations, worded from the questions encountered, and allowing to picture out the joint conditions that it must fulfill:

- First of all, it must enable the impeded thought of a missing general theory of the body in which the so often referred to fantasmatic body could be conceivable while not being reduced to it.
- It must also account for a psychopathological structure of human existence, continuum-spectrum where the crucial experience of corporeity is engaged.
- Finally, it must promise a possible extension of the notion of analyzability to the symptoms yet considered as Actual, which are inseparable from the relational level.

1. As a somatization model, enabling to think the real as well as imaginary body, is missing, the mandatory questions from the body remain unanswered, most of the time, in the concept of actual, which proves an important theoretical shortcoming, unless they are deflected toward an approach which is corrupted from inside by theoretical presuppositions that invariably reduce them to the problem of hysteria. The temptation is thus constant to read the Actual linguistically: François Perrier (Perrier 1978), amongst others authors, recommends the hysterization of hypochondriacs, Ferenczi merely annexes hypochondria into a hysteric structure (Ferenczi 1919). Thanks to this reduction, the issue of the Actual-Neurotic coexistence which is problematic on the clinical level, can be avoided through a suppression of one of the terms at stake. Indeed, Freud already pointed out this synchrony when, he said that actual neuroses were

   more often, however, …intermixed with each other and with a psychoneurotic disorder (Freud 1916–1917, p.390),

   but, that being said, it remains a radical contradiction of his diachronic theoretical conception which simply notes a clinical coexistence! Therefore, even if the resulting missing conceptualization must account for the mechanism operating in the psychoneuroses likely to convey a meaning, it must as well, and as much, not only account for the mechanism operating in the silent and undecipherable symptoms, but also for their coexistence on the clinical level. Where to turn to then, to avoid importing the hysterical model and to go beyond a description which would be untheoretical? We must notice anyway that hysteria provides a result which seems, for a general theory of the body, of major importance: the hysteric's body is the Dream body (Sami-Ali 1987, p.32–33). And yet, what the metapsychology of dream reveals is a continuity relating hypochondria to sleep, to soma, through a common "x", regression to a primary narcissism which can also be understood as well as "normal prototype" of possible morbid conditions (Freud 1915[1917]a, p.222). Then the conceptualization that we intend to discover must identify a background process which plays a major role in the "normal" condition as well as in the "pathological" formations.
2. This first requisite is indeed reinforced with the necessity for the sought concept to point out a psycho pathological structure of human existence, strictly speaking, through which the subject is involved with the world in a very specific relational mode, localized in neurosis, constant in psychosis, and always in

the background of normality. This second condition obviously emerges from the inescapable insistence and from the constancy of the numerous discourses presenting hypochondria as a continuum evolving from normal to pathological around the notion of corporeity in what it brings an intrinsic noncoincidence of the subject with himself and whose anxiety-generating appearance seems an always possible regression to the space of the first objectal relations. On this point, Henri Ey's text (Ey 1950) is meaningful. Beyond the fruitless sleight-of-hand which attempted to equate psychogenesis and sheer mechanisms understood as a curious organo-dynamism, he at least showed how hypochondria, as it asks the eternal question of the "soma-psyche relations," essentially reveals the derealizing function of the body itself which proves that there cannot be any Statics of Real and Imaginary but only perhaps a potential difference, a transmissional tension between two poles. Hypochondria is thus given the status of an illusion, of a "half-reality (Ey 1950, pp.479–480)," representing this ambiguous somatic matter whose dual subject and object existence, dual included and including condition, continually attract us toward anxiety. This continuum then seems superimposable with the one which, in the Freudian corpus, from actual anxiety to psychotic anxiety via all phobiae, describes a spectrum which, wide in its narcissistic dimension, starts with "infra" (actual neurosis) and reaches its climax with "ultra" (narcissistic neurosis): hypochondria, anxiety, narcissism are linked. This ubiquity which highlights the fundamental place of the body in any form of existence only outlines a fact of importance: the reflection on hypochondria causes the Freudian model, qua based on an evolutionary conception, to break up.

3. The conceptualization that we are seeking must finally account for a possible extension of analyzability to the Actual by actualizing its link to transference. But when we situate it as a notion which, confronting the subject to the world, stamps the latter with the mark of unreality and brings the former back to the very first space, we have to face a double epistemological and anthropological problem: an epistemological one, which is the genesis of a representation leading to the very shaping of the very first object; but also an anthropological one, which is the importance of the relational level in this constitution, of the primary nature of this relation which is named "ability to transference". We are also compelled to notice a link of the missing concept with transference if, making good use of the identified analogy between the conception of the theoretical model and the one of the individual libido, and taking into account, in the former, the reshaping fundamentally introduced by the presence of a "hypochondriac complex" subsuming Actual as well as Neurotic, we are still seeking, on an analogical basis again, to establish a possible continuity in the sexual/self-preservation couple. And yet, it seems that it might be their common anchoring in the relational level, for everything, up to the physiological functions, seems to yield to a specific intersubjective context, to a maturing process in a relation to the other person: visual convergence exemplifies it clearly for it is a way of distancing from the maternal face through motivity, so that none of the two partners is annihilated (Sami-Ali 1974, pp.161–196).

What does this mean but that this concept must enable defining the body with this transferential function which shall be clarified, continuum-spectrum composed of the repetitions made possible by the various fixation points, referring to the constitution of functions as well as to the already established functions. Does this mean that this concept seems inseparable from the point of view of the subject as a so-called psychosomatic totality inside which fixation points of different levels can coexist, as actual as well as neurotic facts always happen in a relation to the other? Freud's analysis in front of his friend Fliess, "first preventive cure for paranoia" and occasion of pseudo-cardiac complaints, is indeed the best example of purely transferential Actual symptoms? Freud himself tells it in his Letter n.17:

How sad for a doctor like me who spends every hour of the day to study neuroses to ignore if he is himself affected with a reasonably justified depression or with hypochondria! In such a case we need help··· If you can tell me something certain, please do (Freud 1956, pp.74–76).

Part II
The Obliged Thought

We personally saw the patients mentioned in this study in the Department of Internal Medicine of the Centre Hospitalier de Saint-Germain-en-Laye (France), directed by Dr. Beaufils.

Introduction

Abstract We explain why hypochondria is above all a belief, which relates it to the concept of projection. We also point that clinical observation revealed the cruciality of the concepts of impasse and transference. These reflections lead us to new problematics on the required theoretical model and concepts that will ensure a rigorous and fruitful study of hypochondria.

The operating approach of our first conceptual route is the one of elaboration, "of transition" (Feyerabend 1975, p.202) according to Paul Feyerabend; that is why, this sort of pre-text, can retrospectively look like a paradox. Indeed, to the understanding of a certain type of complaint, devoid of any detectable organic substrate, which is read, in the Freudian system, as possibly hypochondriac, it combines the suspension of evolutionism, the constructive principle which is at the heart of this model: to the chosen approach, conform to clinical experience, of a topical more than chronological gradation which posits as coexisting actual and neurotic phenomena in cases always considered as dual, it applies the usual discourse of the bi-dimensional Freudian model which links simple to complex. This intermediate speech produces nonmeaning and enables a continuum-shaped thought which results in a better posing of the problem and, moreover, gives rise to new problems which are out of reach for Cartesianism. How can we think up a new model which would articulate complex with complex? Can the possible status of transverse notion and the possibility of a projective essence be thought close to this "x" linked to narcissism which is constantly revealed by the continuity of sleep, soma and hypochondria seen as the suffering speech of a totally insomniac body? Counter-induction seems to be the only possible method which provides the perspective of a fundamental conceptual change (Feyerabend 1975, p.21–23).

> We have a point of view (theory, framework, cosmos, and mode of representation) whose elements (concepts, 'facts', pictures) are built up in accordance with certain principles of construction. The principles involve something like a 'closure': there are things that cannot be said, or 'discovered,' without violating the principles (which does not mean contradicting them). Say the things, make the discovery, and the principles are suspended (Feyerabend 1975, p.205).

The violation of the epistemological disconnection established between the concepts of actual and psychoneurotic retrospectively reveals that this disconnection is a belief which was necessary "in advance (Roustang 1976, p.35)." This system, an "obliged thought" (Schneider 1982) analogous to transference, enables a new and possible rationality; it is thus the contradictory background inside which a thinking can take shape and for which several modalities can account: the maternal thought and the necessity to see the unthought in the already-thought, the object of a passion-like relation linking obligation to exclusivity (Aulagnier 1987, pp.174–183), and most notably character formation and its closeness with cultural superego (Sami-Ali 1987, p.19sq). The analysis of this last approach which provides a better intelligibility model will show that the so-called "impeded" thought is only the other side of an "obliged" thought. By analogy with body superego (Sami-Ali 1987, p.65) which says everything that has to be as an anonymous body would, the Freudian somatization model which has actually turned into an ideology seems to be an authoritative vision of the world, a reference framework excluding negativity, dream and subjectivity at the same time. Negativity first: contradiction is unthinkable in a world governed by the logic of likeness so that the norm remains unbreached. What disappears here is the very negativity that thought is made of, replaced by a triumphant redundant positivity. Dream as well: being forbidden, bearing difference, the Imaginary is supplanted by pre-established schemes, rules and categories which come between the subject and the world resulting in a rationality that circumvents obstacles in the name of obviousness. What disappears here is the use of a fundamentally pluralistic methodology that compares ideas to other ideas. Subjectivity at last: to become a second nature, conformation to an external model first evens off everything, reducing the subject to nonexistence in order to exist, this nonexistence being reduplicated by an infinity. What disappears here is the subject himself, to whom an image of reality is substituted, which is a cultural objective of a given society. The reflection on hypochondria cannot avoid the deleterious meeting with what promotes it: ruptures, surges of a displaced speech.

By proposing the title "The obliged thought" we position ourselves from the beginning at the exact points where Freud invited us to go on after him. Some of these points can be recognized: the soma-hypochondria continuity, subsumed in the term of "somatic depression"; the prominent position of this pathology in every place where body image is damaged; the extreme closeness of this problematics to an archaic rupture of the mother-child relationship; the stunning series of multiple denials which specularly link patient and care-giver. But if hypo-chondria can give rise to so many phrases and ways of speaking, if it seems to be the quasi-referential location, the generating focus of so many questionings, what is then the heuristic content of this concept? What specifies it as a problematics? Why does this highly enigmatic aspect give it, above all, the function of a blind spot? As the Freudian model of somatization always leads to the same con-tradictions, we have preferred to study hypochondria on the basis of clinical cases using all those conjoint languages, exploring their limits and their rivalry in order to improve them and to see what concept they can generate.

> Knowledge so conceived is not a series of self-consistent theories that converges toward an ideal view; it is not a gradual approach to the truth. It is rather an ever increasing ocean of mutually incompatible alternatives, each single theory, each fairy tale, each myth is part of the collection forcing the others into a greater articulation and all of them contributing, via this process of competition, to the development of our consciousness (Feyerabend 1975, p.21).

A pluralistic, oneiric and, above all, negative methodology is then adopted. Pluralistic by continuously confronting various registers. Oneiric by trying to break up a conceptual system, which is an image of reality. Negative as it is the thinking of a gap by the adjournment of hierarchical law. Almost anarchistic, Dadaist (Feyerabend 1975, p.12), this thinking constantly points at the extreme contiguity between transference liquidation and delusion, via a specific fantas-matization. Thinking hypochondria but thinking differently: this means ignoring the Freudian fantasy no more, even if it speaks of fantasy a lot...

Chapter 3
Problem Definition

Abstract We clarify two methodological issues. First, in order to overcome the epistemological closure of the Freudian system, closure that hinders the theoretical reflection on hypochondria, we must identify its sticking points. Then, to go beyond them we must not only define the creative but also negative method that we will rely on throughout our study. We explain why we chose to focus on a specific concrete material: the hypochondriac's complaint, in the cases called "negative reports." We explain why this complaint should be studied and interpreted as a discourse, but also in the numerous aspects and levels of the doctor–patient relationship, and as an episode in the hypochondriac's life. The psychosomatic point of view then allows us to formulate hypotheses on how hypochondria articulates to the subject's dynamics and to question the nature of this disorder.

3.1 Object of this Work

Is somatic complaint related to dream as perversion is related to infantile sexual theories? Somatic complaint has an *analogon* of intelligibility that can seemingly be found, in the analytical theory, half-way between hypochondria as an illness of discourse and melancholia as a modality of grief work and an unearthing of one's own cadaver. Could it be related to dream, understood as the par excellence somatic theory in the way Freud explains that its truth comes from its power to provide information in advance on the condition of our organs (Feud 1915[1917]a, p.223), in the same manner as perversion, and particularly fetishism, is to the infantile sexual theories whose "fragment of pure truth" resides in the part of genitality present in infantile sexuality which endow it with an intuition about adult sexuality? This abrupt question represents the polemic direction of development and central hypothesis of this work. It also suggests its deliberate style and method: trying to avoid the etiological perspective, it focuses on "ways of speaking" and conjures up the registers of model and analogy which enable to come close to an order and an economy where an apparent chaos is first seen; they also allow to find an access for the analysis of the relationship that the somatic

M. Derzelle, *Towards a Psychosomatic Conception of Hypochondria*,
DOI: 10.1007/978-3-319-03053-1_3,

complaining patient has with discourse, to reveal meaning in nonmeaning and contradiction, to confront to clinical experience a theoretical elaboration rooted in it and nourished with it, if it is true that

> proposing models is describing by comparison, it is not giving linear causality explanations (Abraham and Torok 1978, p.373).

Ambitious attempt to build a general theory of the body whose problematic absence, so rightly pointed out by J.P. Valabrega (Valabrega 1980, p.15) has undoubtedly affected each phase of this work? Effort to reduce the immeasurable distance between, in the Freudian corpus and even in its last elaborations, the scope of actual neuroses and that of transference neuroses, by means of an analogical line of reasoning which, using imagination to establish a resemblance between what is analyzable and what is not, might reveal the transformation law which turns the anatomical and sexed body into a sexual and metaphorical one, the flesh body as bodily activity and matter into a desiring one as representative activity, the somatic complaint as scientific Unthinkable into an element of dream and thought? Based on positive observation data and nourished on its questionings with a concrete clinical material—the "negative records"—our research resulted in the need for numerous focus shiftings. From this elaboration, a set of rhapsodic notations remains, finally emerged in the "graphic thing"—"coporeal thing" probably too, as something from the body moves into the word and at the same time gives substance. Between knowledge and fantasy, between child and adult, between life and death, on the borderline of analyzability but at the exact painful center of speech, it tries to sketch out a possible intelligibility model of somatic complaint, where the body, far from being held up as a fetish through an excessive positivization, should be related, as well as sex, to the limit which *flaw* or *lack* refer to. Looking for an opening in a category of patients known as unrewarding like hypochondriacs and whose discourse seems to include, in the secret of its cypher, a therapist doomed to fail, sort of lock on the door of the cell where they pay the price of their security.

3.2 What are "Negative Reports"?

As a positive and abstract definition of negative reports would conceal the constant need to consider the interlocutor, doctor, or psychiatrist, to whom the question of naming the illness is asked, it is better to first explain the rule to which they are an exception (differential definition) and tell the communicational twists and turns that lead to them (definition through the relation to the medical community).

We cannot help evoking the circumstances responsible for this interest and this work as an "encounter of the fourth kind." From our often ambiguous position of psychologist-psychotherapist in an Internal Medicine Service, a small hospital department with two units of 30 beds with a certain number of psychiatric patients who could avoid the Psychiatry Unit by being there because their behavior disorders were not too serious, we gradually became conscious of the existence of a fourth kind of somatic symptomatology.

Classically, somatic symptom classification is based, for psychoanalysts as for doctors, psychiatrists, and somaticians, on an opposition that has remained virtually unchanged since the time of Freud, globally setting the existence of three territories. At the two extremes, the etiopathogenic categories are simple: There is either a somatic disease due to a pathogenic factor, affecting the body, or a psychogenic illness, i.e., in which the organs of the body, although possibly algic or inhibited as to the functions, are not affected. The intermediate category, known as psychosomatic, demonstrates the artificiality of this opposition as it combines both organic lesion and psychogenic factor. However, a new idea became obvious: the specular confrontation—due to a request from the medical profession and almost never from the subjects themselves—of these irreducible deviants, unclassifiable and incurable, who are the "sick-who-have-nothing," designated by the Institution under the eloquent name of "negative reports," with this other deviant—"whose fantasy support remains body interdiction" (Fedida 1977a, p.75)—who clearly is the clinical psychologist in a hospital, is undoubtedly part of and contributes to, whenever it takes place, the constitution of a true fourth field of somatic symptoms: that of a speaking-spoken body which, withdrawn from what can be seen and palpated, from what can be shown and demonstrated, demands that be heard, through its complaint and in it, a somatic truth yet denied by the visible representation of the integrity of the said-to-be algic body; that of a body engaged in a language—which names itself with a corporeal synecdoche (Valabrega 1980, p.31)—in which it is represented, as staged, by an organ-centered speech successively worded as topo-logy, patho-logy, and symptomato-logy. But cannot an algy be, precisely, and perhaps above all, a "-logy," and the aches of the soul itself only be expressed in a language that is necessarily the one of the body?

Of course, we do not ignore how arbitrary this dividing line is, even if it is a methodological necessity. First of all, it should be noted that something physiological is usually blended with the most psychogenic and something psychical with the most physiopathological elements,

> analyst and physician both face the gaping lacks of their interpretive system of somatic symptom,

as noted by M.C. Célérier (Célérier 1978). But, above all, what is obvious is the usual coextensivity of the last field with the other three, as somatic complaint is to the patient asking for the doctor's help what the call is to the child asking for the mother's help, in that both address their interlocutor with a speech in which their call can be interpreted.

In the most common cases, diagnosis, that is the intellectual exercise of comparing medical knowledge and somatic complaint, leads, through the possible determination of their intersection locus, to the naming of the disease. Promise of a possible therapeutic as well as implicit conjecture on healing probability and duration, it is the "par excellence" act of, at least verbal, control, amending the patient's relation to his illness in that it shows for him and instead of him what he suffers from in the system of signifiers that constitutes medical discourse, act which contributes to relieving patient anxiety about what he experienced which was not traceable to what could be interpreted from his knowledge on himself, this flow of distressing, painful, stressful, often guilt laden subjective feelings, is included in the medical discourse which assures that a sense can be found in what was previously totally meaningless (Clavreul 1978, p.84).

Diagnosis is usually followed by a reduction in the expression of complaint. In the post-diagnosis period when the patient is given an indubitable existence by the medical profession as the suffering that he expresses and brings is articulable in the signifying components of a syndrome having a place in nosology, it remains on the lowest possible level under the essential form of the expression of a subjectively experienced suffering, undetectable and non-decodable in medical terms. It then matches the "disease of the patient," according to the word of Leriche (Clavreul 1978, p.25), which undoubtedly refers to the only endurable speech on suffering as a state of internal tension bound to end in resolution: background noise of a waiting suffering body.

The less common cases which caught our attention are that of subjects who are qualified "negative reports" at the end of a series of various biological tests, multiple X-ray examinations, repeated auscultations and sophisticated explorations with the conclusion that no medical label could give meaning to the symptoms and no specific etiology or detectable lesion could explain them. If, at first, nothing distinguishes them from "real patients" as they similarly submit to the man of knowledge, from whom they seem to expect both a help and a penalty, a set of complaints and interwoven somatic symptoms, most frequently about cranial or abdominal fixed and persistent pains, on the contrary the somatic complaint that we here face seems to have the function of a challenge to knowledge more than the function of a call. The impossible incorporation of symptoms in medical speech, which is primarily an impossible naming and delimitation by nosology, the resulting absence of therapy except for painkiller prescription, finally the total irreducibility of somatic complaint to silence, which opposes to the nonexistent "medical disease" (the doctor sees nothing) a very present "disease of the patient" (who knows and feels he suffers), all this, in a kind of role reversal, dooms the medical profession to be the frustrating and frustrated bad mother, to be helpless and defeated.

Paradoxically placed in the position of "the one who does not know" in front of someone who holds that what his voice says is more reliable than what his body says, the doctor is invited to recognize, in addition to the possible existence of suffering and pain regardless of any medically recognizable disease—which contradicts the myth of absolute knowledge underlying the assumption of a total understanding of the suffering body—the act of denial on which medical reason is established, as somatic complaint violently recalls that castration cannot be seen if we try to see or represent it. No doubt is that, driven by the dual fear of missing something organic and, on the contrary, of venturing out of the medical system, as Clavreul would say, he first reacts to the aggression which attacks his identity, by, so to speak, taking out his knife: his stabs are called investigations, biopsies and further testings. Part of all the medical hyperactivity so characteristic of the period when, still unknown or poorly known, the disease is the focus of all the interest and desire of the doctor, they give rise to the construction of multiple hypotheses while they constitute a partial answer to the patient's speech, assertion that nothing will be heard that is not objectively verifiable. Attachment and fixation to a symptom, either *cum* or *sine materia*, are likely to be all the more forceful that it has been the cause of an increased or even "armed" interest of the doctor? The question is worth asking. However, when the amount and complexity of the performed explorations oppose the complete absence of conclusive results (with the meaning of "somatically positive"), the persisting discomfort of the ill body is mirrored by the nascent and continuously growing one of the medical "body," the latter term referring both to the doctor's physical body, erogenous and mortal, and to the medical organization, medicine as "immortal" Institution.

Indeed, what does the somatic complainant asks, as he is once again a mere "subject" because of his exclusion from a speech indicating his nonexistence as a patient, and above all subject of the discourse that he has to maintain alone against the medical discourse, that is, against all? One (the doctor), has to give up the visible representation organized by his knowledge and his way of being and to exist as a "look (Sapir 1980, p.7)," to exist as a body hearing what is said of a request which contains love and hatred, repair and destruction, linked together. The other (medicine), has to reject the Act of unawareness which founds it, by admitting its limitations and its non-omnipotence, to exist as a pain hearing that castration is worth an incredible pain which neither seeing nor knowing can be held accountable for. This invitation to replace seeing with hearing and objective with subjective is highly provocative for medical reason. Whereas doctors admit hysterical conversion (which is no acceptable etiology here, for reasons that we will try to expose later) all the more that they use it to explain a form of objective resistance to their interventions, if it is empirically justified by psychosomatic etiology and symptoms in the case of a number of typical syndromes (asthma, allergies, peptic ulcers, etc..), it fundamentally has to be questioned by the hypochondriacal nature or content of a complaint, since it does not obey the rational causality of pain due to a functional disorder or lesion: it would actually be paradoxical for it to tolerate that Somatic, escaping the positive reality of organs and their functions, could become real as an illusion or, somehow, as an Imaginary only experienced in the patient's complaint! Somatic substantiality, instead, is all the more reassuring that the anatomical and pathological representation is and establishes its knowledge through the denial of death and castration, as shown in P. Fedida (Fedida 1971).

What the subject opens up, as he expresses suffering and pain when no diagnosis can be made, is therefore itself a crisis, a sort of "decompensation," putting to question the very foundations of medical identity. It is striking to note how this patient, who sparked a passionate interest in the diagnostic and therapeutic problems he raised, now arouses general hostility. The (somatic) doctor then abruptly declares that he "has nothing" or that "it is nothing" (which means a "somatic negative" indicating the verified normality of the so-called algic organs), or more elegantly sometimes invokes "anorganic," "subjective" or "*sine material*" disorders (all formulations which deny to the subject's body a materiality that only a "beautiful organic disease" could give), but means, in any case, that "it's psychical"—with what this catch-all cliché, which is an eviction, can mean in terms of narcissistic wound, because it is probably precisely to avoid this label that the hypochondriac has long fought with his physical suffering. He then passes the "sick" patient, exhausted by his travel, on to the psychiatrist, sometimes with the secret hope, it seems, that this "psychiatrization" might lead to the symbolic killing of this lamentable "game." Split by the latter, with the meaning of the psychoanalytic concept of splitting (Laplanche and Pontalis 1967, pp.67–69), the doctor also splits him in return, since it is by rejecting the organ-focused complaint that the psychiatrist will try to place it somewhere else, admittedly in a globality, but at the expense of these organs that the investigation identifies as healthy.

"It's psychical." When these words are uttered, usually heard as a denial and a rejection into the lower class, the one of imagination and subjectivity, rather than as a possible expansion of the horizon to consider, the second act of the tragic dialogue opens; its major protagonist, taking over from the somatic doctor, is the psychiatrist. His characteristic is, for us, that he repeats the same seemingly sado-masochistic sequence as the one previously mentioned, arousing the same helpless response and ending, again as the previous sequence, with a dismissal, as no naming of the presented symptoms is possible. Rupture and continuity here go hand in hand. Subject of a seesaw movement from (negative) somatic to (possibly positive) psychic, one of the actors of the drama has withdrawn behind the scenes, but the patient who never ceases to proclaim his suffering constantly performs the same play again and again. The outcome is identical, denial of the "bad" which occurs in the form of a reparation gift and that the complainant can only, in turn, interpret radically as a withdrawal effect. A specific structure of communication thus gradually emerges from the relationship, whose watchwords are repetition and reduplication. Because somatic complaint seems to have the power of arousing an impotent response, melting pot of an imaginary twinning and of a mirroring symmetrization where the other person functions as a necessary projection of frustration. The mechanism is simple. What the psychiatrist imaginarily tends to identify with is the idealized maternal ego in the patient's complaint. This iden-tification leads him to speak and act in the ideal auto-gratifying representation of the good object. Frustrating the patient by his verdict as it is negative, he is, like the "bad mother," frustrated by him in return since he is held dependent on his inability to be everything. The patient depersonalizes the other person to reduce him to the anonymous and impersonal medium of the internal instance, that, by projection, he entrusts him with. Projective identification is at work, coupled with a sort of retro-projection. This might suggest the hypothesis of a pathogenesis related to primary narcissistic organization.

What happens when this subject whose symptoms, although disabling, always remain very mundane, meets the psychiatrist is quite surprising. Considering the somatic complaint, or rather its discordance with bodily integrity, as a nosographic entity or as the expression of a given structure would certainly be nonsense. As it is the case for anorexia, alcoholism and bulimia, the precision and simplicity of the symptomatic boundaries have indeed for corollary an infinitely wide definition in the field of reference structures, which eventually covers the entire nosography (Igoin 1979, p.131)?

On the contrary, it is surprising to notice the lack of attempts to identify the possible modalities that could address the issue of somatic complaint with no detectable organic substrate. It is true that there are many possible paradigms: hysteria with its polymorphic pains when there is no real injury, hypochondria and its imaginary ailments leading to etiological research behaviors and call for medical help, depression and its close somatic equivalents in Psychiatry textbooks (Griesinger, Esquirol) in the chapter on hypochondria, melancholy and the rehashing of a complaint which has the meaning of a grieving process. What we have here is therefore less a symptom than a sign, experienced differently according to the psychical economy within which it takes place. We must however immediately stress that, in the cases that we encountered, labeled "negative reports," one of the four proposed paradigms cannot be effectively maintained: that of hysteria. If certain personality traits sometimes show its very specific defense arrangements, the main characteristics of the reported disorders indeed seem to have nothing in common with it, as evidenced by their monotony and banality. Fixed and persistent, truly haunting, and focused on a single territory, they point-by-point oppose the usually moving and floating symptomatology of the "beautiful indifferent." From its beginning, the relationship with the medical profession neither mitigates nor displaces them. Previous medical history reveals neither repetition nor possible migration and metamorphosis. Their mode of expression, influenced by the extent of genuine suffering, gives rise to no drama. Neither displacements nor metaphors, that is why they show some analogy with these senseless symptoms that Freud mentioned about actual neuroses (Freud 1916–1917, p.385). More exactly, unlike the primary meaning of neurotic symptoms, they only have a secondary meaning, acquired after the fact, and have not triggered the symptom formation process.

Should we consider a certain "anti-hypochondria" of the psychiatrist, appearing as the very expression of his medical vocation, as the cause of his persistent preference for negative report diagnoses rather than hypochondriacal ones? Like his fellow somatic doctors, he seems to agree with a conception of hypochondria viciously based on a reference to the materiality of the fact which motivates the complaint. Even Freud did not escape this mirage. Assuming that it was material, he wrote:

> hypochondria must be right, organic changes must be present in it. But what could these changes be (Freud 1914, p.83)?

His answer is well-known: erogeneity. Note that this typically medical way to ask whether the patient is "wrong" or "right" reveals, in the first case, a manifest prejudice against hypocondria, based on the concept of *sine materia* disease, and in the second case, a just as aggressive connivance with the disease, where the psychiatrist's own hypochondria is unmasked, "Doctor Despite Himself," but "Imaginary Invalid"[*] indeed! In both cases, an identification occurs. The "meeting of two narcissisms" is probably better tested and known by the psychiatrist than by his interlocutor: he knows that it implies a lethal risk as when Narcissus names himself recognizing himself in the fountain, "Iste ergo sum," the poet's Hero shouts (Ovid, *Metamorphoses*, III, 463). But the psychiatrist refuses to utter this fatal Word. Also, preferring to admit his ignorance, he says: "I do not understand what it is," "I do not see."

3.3 A Guiding Thread: The Register of Hypochondria

Now that we have identified and joined the emerging keystones in order to understand the nature of the register of negative reports, the general meanings appear. In the first place, and unlike medical discourse, the discourse of the somatic complainant brings nothing to mind, at least nothing visible. In line with the formulation of the theoreticians of Palo Alto which states that each human behavior can be considered as a game, a communication process, where people communicate and metacommunicate to influence the other, we can therefore say that negative reports belong to the category of never ending games, patient and doctor being both stuck in a communicational double impasse, a "double bind" difficult to break. Game of the patient who may have nothing and the doctor who sees nothing, where a double blindness is involved: that of the doctor who sees nothing where the patient tells him that there is something and that of the patient who tries to suggest the existence of a conflict but who does not see at all. In Winnicott's terms, the establishment of such a dialogue would be characterized by the nonoverlapping of the intermediate personal areas of the two subjects, one trying to make the other accept the objectivity of its subjective phenomena. Specifically, with the closing of a speech that the other cannot understand in the absence of a third term belonging to a shared external reality, one could say that the patient, by an internalization of the transitional space, keeps using his inside "as the whole symbolic space (Calligaris 1987, pp.53–63)." Two speeches meet, but each is revealed to the other as the place where a response arises whose validity cannot be guaranteed by a third instance: the analogy with psychotic speech is obvious.

After this observation of a "double link" relationship, which is also a relationship "around nothing" since the object does not exist as such, we can notice its repetitive aspect. Paradoxically attracting the attention of many caregivers in spite of the banality of his symptoms, the patient indeed repeats, with each care professional, the same sequence of behavior organized in the same phases. Therefore, the only real issue seems to be the fact that the somatic complainant finally finds the evidence, thanks to this kind of mirror-witness and bad mother, that the medical profession knows nothing more than he does. In Kleinian terms, this continual need for the patient to confirm his omnipotence by the repeated testing of the masochism of the other person, would be referred to as the manic position. If it helps fight depressive anxiety (Kein 1968, p.346), the use to manic-type defenses is above all a refuge from paranoid situations that are difficult to control (Klein 1968, p.327), especially in front of the fear inspired by internalized persecutors like the parental couple for example. Intimately related to ambivalence because it implies a necessary identification to the bad objects, at the same time as a negation of the terror they generate, omnipotence then enables the young child's ego, but also the adult's when he operates at the most archaic level, to assert himself, to a certain extent, in the face of his internal persecutors. Due to the absence of more suitable means to effectively deal with guilt and anxiety, manic defense is therefore closely linked with obsessive defense: the repeated failures of the subject's attempts of reparation push his ego to use an alternate mechanism. From this point of view, therefore, in the negative reports, the question of naming the illness arises again and again: the measure of the triumph over the bad internal objects, which is a function of the impotence found in the other person, depends on it. This undoubtedly generates, between the medical profession and the patient who claims to be ill, an impressive set of negations and counter-negations, where, having again indicated the primitive nature of the problem suggested, we can finally stress the importance of the negativist attitude in the somatic complainant's discourse. Because, opposing the "nothing" of the doctor's conclusion, the "something" which gains its knowledge from failure, is an essentially positive act that the patient performs, in a defense movement. "Something rather than nothing." Like this famous formula, which in short is the fetishist's motto, invites us to think, it even seems to be a denial. Could then negative reports be one of the possible fates of the perverse *Spaltung*? Things are more complex. Certainly, as the fetishist, the somatic complainant cancels and approves at the same time a knowledge on reality, namely all the more ambiguous that its object is an absence (absence of disease here echoing absence of the mother's penis' in the mentioned perversion): he knows that there is "nothing" medically speaking but continues to believe that he has "something." While the fetishist uses the object to replace the missing word, as G. Rosolato explains it in his analysis of the case mentioned by Freud (Rosolato 1978, p.27), on the contrary negative reports seem to use words to replace things, words which then become the real location of bodily modification. In other words, if "the object takes over from the words" for the former, this order is inverted for the latter: the logic of discourse only matters, words being really treated as things. This results in this paradoxical situation where the condition of organs only fits the words actualized in complaint, speech becoming the only possible projective surface of the somatic. Denying the denial of medical discourse is thus a way for the patient to provide the so-called algic organ with the eternity of a presence only finally consisting in the verbal delusion of it in his speech. "Something is something" is then cynically valid word for word. We mean that

the predominance of what has to do with words over what has to do with things (Freud 1915, p.200),

provides the organ with a representation in thought on the basis of an analogy or identity of verbal expression; in this very formula we can easily recognize, apart from the one of schizophrenic speech, the formation process of speech.

Hypochondria: it is for us a guiding thread, a sort of privileged reference, which seemed appropriate both in our attempt at analyzing the patient-physician relationship and in our own encounters with patients in the interviews requested by the medical profession in times of crisis. Our use of this register as a modality for a possible reading of negative reports is not to be understood as diagnostic, even less as structural; our purpose is certainly not to say that we are in the presence of hypochondriacs. We rather formulate the assumption that the coexistence, in the psychic economy of the encountered patients, of large non-elaborated areas and neurotic problems—with the same meaning as when, speaking of actual neuroses in his *Introduction to psychoanalysis*, Freud said

> more often, however, they are intermixed with each other and with a psychoneurotic
> disorder (Freud 1915, p.200),

and we then use hypochondria as paradigm and theme. Other ways, involving other figures, are also possible. Here are some of them: perversion, depression, mania, melancholy. On these different milestones, this dimension however has the advantage of taking into account the general meanings of the patient−physician relationship, and to articulate the most critical aspects of the somatic complaint with no detectable organic substrate. Three of them are worth being highlighted:

(1) Negative report essentially consists in a discourse which questions other discourses which call themselves "curing," since the symptomatology is there merged in the patient's language. The proximity of hypochondria as a disease of speech must then be considered.

(2) Rather than a state, a negative report is a sort of nodal point, a tipping point often just a little ahead of the onset of the disease. According to, in the aftermath, the experience of the medical profession, the frequent morbid evolution in the form of serious organic or psychological disorders (cancer, delusional episode, etc.) retrospectively indeed means that, like dream (Freud 1915[1917]a, p.221), it has positive diagnostic capacities, and that it is the historical precedent of the symptoms of multiple diseases to come. We therefore recognize here, extended to the organic pathology, the overall Freudian formulation of the temporal articulation of Actual with Neurotic, especially the one of hypochondria with different psycho-pathological forms, at the forefront of which paranoia lies, in its intimate dependency with an underlying theory of the suffering body (Freud 1973a, p.368).

(3) Finally, all the atypical symptoms of negative reports mainly seem characterized by their monotony and banality, qualities which are the very same as the uniform affect of anxiety neurosis (Freud 1973b, p.21). Undoubtedly, in a number of cases, its somatic equivalents happen to feed concerns in a shift from the outside to the inside.

Our work is thus constantly connected, from side to side, with the dimension of the ACTUAL. What is however exactly expressed with this term designating a group of neuroses somehow located, in the Freudian corpus, on the fringe of psychoanalysis? It is here that our interest awakens, the recourse to hypochondria inviting, as in return, to question the register in which it fits.

Chapter 4
Negative Reports or "A Certain Discourse Used in a Certain Way"

Abstract Clinical observation allows us to identify invariants in hypochondriacal discourse. We notice that they belong to three categories that we define and interpret. In terms of content, complaint is characterized by a meaningful location of the said-to-be algic part of the body. The psychological aspects are mainly a tendency to conflict euphemization, a specific dynamic of depressive and paranoid traits and a basal fantasy inhibition. However, our interpretation of the centrality of complaint and the intensity of discourse experience, as well as the inevitable therapeutical failure in hypochondria induce new hypotheses.

4.1 Stories, Briefly Told

After the failure of the psychiatrist called to the rescue as the specialist of the invisible soul, the first medical action is to send the patient to the psychologist. The invariability of the moment when this happens is to highlight, which seems to endow this demand with the aim of repressing unconscious fantasies, specific to the department, which the somatic complainant has progressively revealed. It is in this context that we have worked on negative reports, in interviews which sometimes had limited possibilities because the discharge date was close. In a number of cases yet, we could continue our task in the form of weekly outpatient interviews which unquestionably enabled the accomplishment of real work, which even "resulted" in the displacement of a patient's symptoms. We will try to draw the main features of these very dissimilar fates that are stories above all.

The four exposed cases relate to apparently quite ordinary people whose common point is, beyond their various individual issues, that they express pain and suffering while no diagnosis can be made. More exactly, if it is true that, as M. C. Célérier writes.

physical suffering, even the most hysterical or hypochondriac one, must have a physical substratum, at least a microchemical one (Célérier 1978, p.131),

M. Derzelle, *Towards a Psychosomatic Conception of Hypochondria*,
DOI: 10.1007/978-3-319-03053-1_4,
© Springer International Publishing Switzerland 2014

these patients have first and foremost the characteristic of expressing a somatic complaint with no detectable organic substrate. Let us then make their words audible, words they uttered in laborious interviews whose grueling aspect evokes the accurate picture depicted by M. Balint when he speaks of complaint with a general meaning.

> True, we do not give our patient – as doctors do – sedatives, tranquilizers, anti-depressants, and other drugs, but perhaps this makes it more difficult for us to bear unrelieved complaints. To be able to do something about them, to give something to stop them, we resort to giving interpretations, and if these do not stop the complaining, we try to fix the blame somewhere: on ourselves for our bad technique, on the patient for his incurable illness, for his destructiveness, his deep regression, for the split in his ego, and so on; or on his environment, and in particular on his parents for their lack of understanding, their unsympathetic ways of upbringing, and so on; recently an old scapegoat seems to have been resuscitated for this purpose: heredity. In this way, an endless spiral may develop... however no real change follows (Balint 1967, p.109).

4.1.1 Case I

Mrs. C., aged 40, entered the hospital on her attending physician's advice, but this hospitalization also seemed to be her desire. She had been feeling very tired for a while and she presently suffered from pains, described as steady and shooting, in the left hypochondrium; for a certain time those pains had been related to gynecological problems which had been taken care of. Except for a light and varying anemia occasionally revealed by her blood count, nothing noticeable could be reported. Her previous medical history only revealed an eczema episode when she was four and benign adenopathies in childhood. She had decided to see her doctor because she had felt dizzy once, and only once, a few weeks before; she attributed her dizziness to the obstinacy of her pains which she said were beginning to completely exhaust her. After multiple investigations, Mrs. C. apparently had nothing thinkable from a medical point of view.

When we met her for the first time, Mrs. C. told us, smiling brightly, that she had never had any psychological problem. She was a management executive in an advertising company, she looked much younger than her age and, apart from her illness on which she was unstoppable, she was only fluent and comfortable when speaking about her job. Giving a lot of technical details and pointing insistingly at the form of independence it provided her, she described it as very absorbing and demanding. She had divorced 3 years ago by mutual agreement with her ex-husband, because of "weariness" she said. She said that this separation was an inevitable fatality, because, as in all couples habit soon replaces affection. During this marriage, she had had a miscarriage after 7 months of pregnancy before giving birth to a stillborn child; those events seemed to have influenced the divorce but the patient did not say much about this. After her divorce Mrs. C. began a Bachelor's Degree in Economic Sciences and then brilliantly obtained it, more to prove to herself that she could achieve something than because of genuine necessity. However she mentioned a lot of difficulties in her present work. As a sort of permanent backdrop, an "implausible fatigue" had been crushing her for a few months; she said that it was the result of a sleeplessness caused by noisy neighbors. Recent holidays had not helped her recover as she still had difficulties to fall asleep. In spite of a growing exhaustion, she had continued to work until dizziness and pain had appeared. Now on sick leave she was pleased to think that the cause of her problems would be identified but strongly deplored her "idleness."

Interviews with Mrs. C. were, on the whole, extremely difficult: when she was invited to talk about herself, she tirelessly returned either to very general considerations or to an endless inventory of her internal somatic condition, as bodily life and medical prescriptions were obviously the only objects of her attention of the moment. Cold and aloof, she seemed to undergo a sort of police interrogation in which she would have had to cunningly dodge questions. All this, marked by the incessant to-ing and fro-ing of considerable paranoid anxieties alternately related to the inside, the body, (hypochondriac persecutions) and coming back from the outside where they had been projected (paranoid persecution), identified her as basically depressive, register to which the continuously expressed fatigue and sleep disturbance also pertained. Shortly before she left the hospital, Mrs. C. "confessed" that she sometimes felt "depressed" and would then have done "anything" but she was violently trying to defend herself against this suffering by a haughty attitude in the relationship similarly to her choice of an unbridled hyperactivity at work.

Manifested above all by a radical economic transformation of investments, the depression of Mrs. C. essentially appeared to us in perfect match with the notion of somatic depression proposed by P. Fedida (Fedida 1978b, p.76), as it seemed to share a genuine structural isomorphism with organic disease: same interest and libido withdrawal from objects in the outside world, same concentration of those on the so-called algic organ, in short, same narcissistic reorganization strongly auto-eroticized by the organic pains and suffering and economically protected by the patient's somatic selfishness, with the difference that, in the second case,

the painful sensations are based on demonstrable changes.

There is no doubt therefore that this is an absolute "regression" in the topical and temporal meaning of the term (Laplanche and Pontalis 1967, pp.400–401), primitive narcissism being precisely considered by Freud as the sleeper's and the somatic patient's as well, but also as the hypochondriac's.

The psychical state of a sleeping person is characterized by an almost total withdrawal from the surrounding world and a cessation of all interest in it (Freud 1915[1917]a, p.222),

formulation repeated in identical terms in *On Narcissism: An Introduction* when he speaks of organic disease before coming to hypochondria (Freud 1914, p.83sq). The depression-soma-sleep-hypochondria continuity seems to emerge, already suggested by the ancients, like Griesinger, in the form of a community of structure between hypochondria and depression named somatic neurasthenia. Mrs. C. thus seems, like the organic patient, to entrust her somatic evolution with the function of resolving the deadlock generated by her conflicts. The alternation noted by Freud between cessation of love life (withdrawal from object libido) and onset of disease (narcissistic libido) goes in the same direction, suggesting specific correlations between the two processes (Freud 1914, p.89). As somatic illness, the depressive state of Mrs. C. perhaps tells the disaster of a breakup.

4.1.2 Case II

Mrs. P., aged 39, entered the Department in a panic, for a right cranial pain that was precisely located at the level of the parietal bone; she was determined and asked for a CT scan in order to know what this "concealed." As a former medical student, she feared brain damage and exposed to anybody available her multiple reasons to suspect a serious pathology. Very accurately, she described a fixed and persistent painful "point," which she had suffered from, without climax or respite, for approximately 5 months, more precisely since her second delivery. Shortly before, she said, she had developed large scalp furuncles in the same location, now healed as the dermatologist called to her bedside rapidly confirmed it. Having, in her words, never experienced the single headache, she expressed her astonishment especially at being overwhelmed by pain, and tirelessly denounced the "remarkable weakness" of all "lame and pale" descriptions that the medical profession in vain tried to make to "perhaps" identify her problem. Strictly speaking, for her, the typical matter seemed, to be the Inexpressible and the Elusive. Convinced of being able to be understood only very approximately, she seemed in this to match Freud's description of the hypochondriac evoking his pain:

> the neurasthenic... (a hypochondriac or a person affected with anxiety neurosis) gives the impression of being engaged in a difficult intellectual task to which his strength is quite unequal (...). He struggles to find a means of expression. He rejects any expression of his pains proposed by the physician even if it may turn out afterwards to have been unquestionably apt. He is clearly of opinion that language is too poor to find words for his sensations and that those sensations are something unique and previously unknown of which it would be quite impossible to give an exhaustive description. For this reason he never tires of constantly adding fresh details, and when he is obliged to break off he is sure to be left with the conviction that he has not succeeded in making himself understood by the physician (Freud 1892–1895, p.136).

If there was, for Mrs. P., the equivalent of a double imaginary lesion, that of her brain echoing that of the medical ideal which had guided her once, investigations, often made on her request, did not however reveal anything abnormal. Then, labeled 'negative report," Mrs. P. could leave the hospital after 10 days.

When we met Mrs. P., we were struck by her physical appearance. Livid and tired, her face lit up with an indescribable smile, as soon as she spoke of herself, a little as if she was injured and endured in silence an inner suffering whose evocation would be forbidden. Her story also constantly presented her in a victim role.

When she was 8-years old she had contracted poliomyelitis, as a result, according to her, of a vaccination error—which would have consisted in the inoculation of a stale product—but fortunately had no real handicap due to this condition, and she ceaselessly returned to the subject of this painful period of her existence. And the feeling, experienced very early, to be different from the others because of being "ill" occupied center stage. The evocation of this exceptional status made her immediately associate with the immense fatigue she said she had felt since the birth of her second child. She sometimes connected her cranial pain to this birth. Her second child, a girl, was however desired, especially by her because, she added "my husband already had his boy." Recently however, fatigue had begun to make her nervous and sometimes she could not withstand her husband, her 3-year-old son either, whom she admitted, with a deep feeling of guilt, she had intended to hit many times. She also explained that in the past, and especially just after her marriage, the relationship with her husband, nice but very choleric, "tolerating no single moment of resistance," had frequently been difficult and marked by a lot of violence. As she understood that her husband took "a certain pleasure" in such quarrels, she then tried to avoid them and not to respond to provocations. "Someone had to give in!" she said then, faintly giving her unruffled smile. Mrs. P. also spoke of many difficulties in her professional life. Having given up, after 5 years, medical studies that were "prodigiously boring and not a life for a woman," she had folded back on pharmacy, learning the job of pharmacy technician. Her boss supposedly had recently threatened to dismiss her for having added her month's holiday, without warning him, to her legal maternity leave. The patient seemed to accept this fact as inevitable and did not even consider the big financial problems, which would undoubtedly arise if she lost her job.

In this story repeatedly marked by the dimension of failure and suffering, the most prominent feature was the resigned, nearly submissive, attitude, of Mrs. P. toward the private and social conflicts of her existence. Invariably, at work as well as in her couple, she seemed to find herself in the position of the one who must withstand and remain silent, the one especially who, without having the means to respond, constantly has to face the aggression and violence of the other person. It is also without a word or reaction that she endured, as blows of destiny, the multiple external frustrations apparently tirelessly imposed by reality and external circumstances. No doubt we can therefore as a first approximation think that this docile and submissive attitude in which she seemed to be frozen, which is entirely subjection and passivity was very early rooted in our patient in the early experience of her illness, real *fatum* and injustice of destiny, probably felt as such. However, if we leave the point of view of the object for the one of the subject, the prevailing and determining role of frustration seen as internal is revealed to us in a very blatant way, Mrs. P. clearly refusing, as the result of fixation or internal conflicts, all forms of satisfaction that reality could offer. At this level, it was the effective satisfaction of her own desire, the satisfaction of her own drive demands that the patient refused to herself. And finally, less than the impossibility to receive a satisfaction of any kind, it was the response to a specific requirement involving a mode of satisfaction that is at stake. We must invoke the notion of moral masochism is necessary here, Mrs. P. seeking above all the victim position, be it indiscriminately imposed.

> by someone who is loved or by someone who is indifferent is of no importance. It may even be caused by impersonal powers or by circumstances.

What she reported of the relationship with her husband resembled a sado-masochistic relationship. What can we also say about this child desired by her and which is placed as a counterpoint to the boy now destined to the desire of the father? What to say, again, of these medical studies so suddenly stopped for the benefit of a profession surprisingly chosen with no consideration for her intellectual capacities? What can we finally say about the incredible situation that she stuck herself into at work? Frank expression of self-punishment? As if it were to continue unabated a certain amount of suffering, a form of "pain" coming to be relayed by another, Mrs. P. seemed to strive to counter, one by one, each of her personal desires and withstood these repeated frustrations putting herself in the position of good-mother-good-wife, position that the birth of a second child had once again revealed in its binding necessity. However, aggressiveness against the other person sometimes resurfaced, and on this occasion the urge to hit her son emerged, sort of secondary reversal of the masochistic drive.

Under these circumstances, we feel that a plural reading of her somatic symptom should be made with various modalities which should all refer to an essentially narcissistic problem. It probably revived, for Mrs. P., the issue of body image already so painfully affected by her previously contracted disease, thus forcing her somehow to take care of herself exclusively, for once. The symptom was therefore also, presumably, a demand for recognition as a desiring subject, request already expressed in her desire to have a child "for herself" but never implemented or heard. From this perspective, the body would therefore be the only place where something like desire could come again to be meant, albeit in a language remaining forever incomprehensible. It is however primarily as an exact repetition of a sado-masochistic scenario originally formed around organic disease and frequently replayed since then in many intersubjective conflicts that this somatic symptom deserves to be located. Subscribing to the words of M.C. Célérier on the double somatic and psychic connection of fantasy, we can indeed apply them literally to the case currently outlined, as we think that somatic symptoms should always be linked to the subject's life history and structure in the same way as psychic symptoms. As

> any symptom affecting the body, regardless of its most obvious cause, is for the psychic field charged with some sense and strength. This strength both depends on the importance of body damage and on the economic organization of the psyche. The meaning of the symptom is conferred by its occurrence at a time in the history of the subject for which the psychic representations have already been linked to the experienced body. For the subject, it refers to the representative fantasies of the sexual or identificatory conflict that the disease brings to the foreground, fantasies inscribed in the elective attachment points of his personal background (Célérier 1978, pp.122–123).

As such, it is interesting to point that Mrs. P. invariably traced the origin of her pain to the birth of her daughter, via the brief organic interlude constituted by the furuncle episode. This explanatory attempt, amazing in the words of a former medicine student was part of an effort to rationalize a painful somatic condition whose etiology was to be found somewhere else. But it was illuminating about the possible secondary meanings that the patient could give to this regression to a hypochondriac behavior that had precisely led her to be taken in charge, as when she was a child, by doctors. Infantile sex theory referring to a possible begetting from the head similarly to the "delivery of ideas"? Projection of a paranoid nature of the bad object to the limit of the outside and inside just before its hypochondriac re-introjection into the body? Reuse of the symptom provided by reality as representative of unconscious fantasies waiting for an opportunity to manifest itself? Classic fantasy of the hypochondriac register? The numerous interpretations "after the fact" of the symptom are as many sense injections conveying above all the subject's life history and structure.

4.1.3 Case III

Mr. C., 26 years, of southern origin, was hospitalized in the service for 2 weeks to undergo a complete check up on the advice of his doctor. In recent months, he had ceaselessly complained of a persistent abdominal pain with neither identifiable rhythmicity nor notable triggering factor, as well as of an intractable left hemicranial pain. Despite multiple explorations, no specific etiology had been found and it was obviously with great concern about this inability to name the symptoms that Mr. C. apprehended and asked for hospitalization. All previous treatments had remained without effect and, very puzzled, the patient reported on several occasions the strange diagnosis of "digestive tetany" advanced during an examination by a radiologic technologist. During the first visit of the doctors to his room, while he itemized and discussed very carefully each of his symptoms, his wife, present, participated very actively although silently to the description being done, imperturbably nodding with a terribly anxious expression. Although it was somewhat daring to say so so early, Mr. C.'s symptoms especially seemed to have a real importance in the functioning of its couple. Another remarkable fact: to each caregiver, Mr. C. repeated the detailed story of his illness, in almost identical terms and in a neutral tone. Presenting his symptoms not as an expression of pain but as a sort of riddle instead; he said that he understood nothing about it but entirely trusted the medical team.

During the interviews that we could have with him, apart from his symptoms, his daily life, with all its banality, occupied center stage. He was currently a police officer and he declared that he loved his job even if he had initially intended to be a lifeguard on the beaches, position for which he had been rejected twice, he did not tell us why. He had married shortly after his transfer to Paris 4 years before and had no child. In spite of our questions Mr. C. very tersely described some vague childhood memories only telling their factual elements. Until the age of seven, he had spent most of his time with his family in Morocco where his father had been assigned. This man had died of throat cancer shortly after the family's return to France, leaving a very large family whose youngest child was 3-months old. According to the patient, there was nothing traumatic however in this and he only spoke about very mundane things. When we prompted him to evoke the death of his father, he vaguely seemed to overcome emotion but the affect visibly did not stick to the words. Obviously, the sudden reminding of this event suddenly induced the urgent need to adopt as much as possible the position of witness/look which he imagined was his interlocutor's. Thus, he very occasionally gave the impression of reproducing the mirrored psychic activity that, by splitting and projection probably, he seemed to assign to the other person, in a representation of himself through the representation that he had of his counterparts. When speaking about the death of his father, his tone remained neutral, and he even concluded adding: "he had to, that's all!" Similarly, speaking of his sister who had had an arm damaged by poliomyelitis, an "incident": "there are many others who have surely had worse!" Finally, referring to the potential danger of his job, he said: "must not think about it!" What was surprising therefore about Mr. C. was, according to him, the total absence of problems, which could be the negation of conflictualization. The events that could have raised anxiety or caused pain seemed cast aside. Mr. C. insisted however on his good adaptation to Parisian life. At work as in his family he underlined the way that he got along perfectly with everyone. He therefore declared that he was for the moment fairly satisfied with his life, his desire being expressed as exclusively modeled according to the desire of the Other, another who would not be intended as relational but rather as social, collective and impersonal. Due to a discourse giving the impression to register as a veneer of conventions, interviews with Mr. C. were extremely difficult, or even challenging. In such a relationship indeed, the other person is finally just there to justify and reinforce what can perhaps be called a feeling of static control of reality, of psychic reality first and foremost. The discomfort experienced facing patients of this type can be connected to the nonperception of authentic affect, as if symbolization was suddenly emptied of all its value. In the case of Mr. C., the only thing that could be addressed, at least, under the sign of conflict, was thus paradoxically the symptom, "the riddle." As he liked to repeat, he wanted to "do away" with his symptoms but, at the same time, he wondered with some fear if anything "bad" could be found. This ambivalence seemed important to us as it was the place of a contradiction which, for Mr. C. could neither be said nor take shape. Only evoked but visibly very distant from any conscious elaboration, it was yet in a remarkable proximity since his body was at stake. However conflict itself was probably the real issue of this contradiction, conflict that Mr. C. precisely strove, and by all means, to hold off. Here, symptom was above all a sort of nodal point from which the confrontational aspects of his life could emerge. A riddle that he questioned but found no answer to. In doing so, it nevertheless remained for a considerable time the focusing point of the subject's interest, sign or at least paradigm of a conflict center which, as it could not be heard elsewhere, was inscribed in the body. Even if such an interpretation can be questioned we cannot help proposing it, as the somatic symptoms of Mr. C. irresistibly suggest some sort of equivalent or substitute for a specific questioning having found no other practicable routes than those of the body.

We can finally add that, as it was basically a-symbolic, the case of Mr. C. evokes by many sides what P. Marty and M. de M'Uzan described in operational behavior and thought as essential depression, when they noted the frequency of its installation shortly before the outbreak of multiple diseases. In the first place, the "banal" and "consistent" character of a speech which very significantly over-invests current and factual reality within a relationship that is particularly dry and strongly marked by the weight of necessity, is to highlight, in a close match with the traditional description of the critical point of any progressive disorganization:

> Representations are poor, repetitive, marked by the seal of current and factual aspects. The patient proceeds automatically, without insight, by presenting the actuality of his imme-diate symptoms, failing to consider either his own depressive state or the globality of his individuality and the experienced context. The word seems to be deprived of its substance, reduced almost to a vocal activity expressing facts, and seemingly rudimentary affects and representations, concerning some realities of the time. Subject to certain aspects of the outside reality in which he remains inserted in many ways, with no possibilities of internal distancing from the outside, with no prospect of mobilizing his status or that of other people, thus with no hope of adaptation, with no desires or pleasures, however exposed to injuries and diseases, the subject of operational life often suggests the image of a living dead (Marty 1980, pp.95–99).

In fact, the main characteristic of meetings with Mr. C. was the lack of sponta-neity, the absence of dramatization of speech, as if, far from repressing any fantasy activity but rather being the prey of the fantasy of being reduced to an external representation, he chose to show only what in fact was a façade, a lack perhaps, in the form of a defensive fetishization of the Somatic. However, this *status quo* does absolutely not resist investigation and very quickly, the ideic banality of the story appeared, as a kind of way to stop time and life in their fundamentally disruptive movement, in all likelihood so as to provide the Ego, through this totally static control, with a position seen as more comfortable in that it always remains true to form. Secondly, when we highlight a reduplication in the relationship, inseparable from a true psyche-soma splitting, it is not without mentioning, as in essential depression, a pathogenesis related to the primary narcissistic organization. If the latter indeed seems to evoke a regression corresponding to an installed fixation at the level of the anaclitic depression described by R. Spitz (Spitz 1965), the allocation, by projection of any psychic activity on another person (therapist, wife, etc.) sim-ilarly seems to reproduce here an extremely archaic rupture occurred in the exchange with the maternal body or environment. Perhaps this somatic-psychic rupture is related to a possible failure of the specular relationship to the mother's body and so to that to the intermediate area where, according to Winnicott, creativity and play take place. The apparent inability of the patient to "fantasize," to find a word from and based on an "area of illusion," then evokes the time of the outset of trauma, as the rupture basically relates to what happens between mother and child. It can then be assumed that, in this traumatic situation, the child has structured a particular splitting identifying all his psyche to his mother that factually reflects her image and no other. When Mrs. G. repeated, dramatizing it, the nonverbalized fear of her husband, what did she do but perform a sort of "translocation" that we can call compensatory, re-elaborating his unspoken feelings?

4.1.4 Case IV

Mrs. B., age 52 was hospitalized for a week in the service, complaining of severe abdominal pain for which she had already undergone multiple explorations. For almost 2 years, she had had a painful area that she could very accurately locate, revealing her abdomen and pointing her right index finger between the left hypochondrium and the pit of the stomach. At the request of different doctors, she had already undergone an impressive amount of examinations including countless X rays, designating all the medical as an art being first of all a clairvoyance. Pyelography study, ultrasounds, cholecystography, endoscopies, laparotomies, small intestine, and colon transit study, as well as exercise and resting electrocardiograms were thus performed, all negative; their manifest cascading series seems close to the description made by H. Maurel of the unlawful inspection requested by the hypochondriac to the doctor:

> He wants to see, to be seen, and to see himself watched. He shows off his body to see himself in the eyes of the other person. Without shame, skirts are spontaneously lifted, the successive shells of underwear and girdles are hastily stripped to denude the suffering body, the painful belly, the skin offered to medical palpation, the orifices that reveal to the clinician the natural entrances to the depths of the body. But, beyond the specular image of a skin envelope, beyond the disappointing mirror, what the patient desires is introspection. That is the reason of his recourse to the competence of the other person, whose piercing and inquiring gaze creeps beyond a simple surface inspection, to the dark lair of entrails, by subtle break-in techniques. So begins the adventure of wonderful endoscopies, made using instruments, penetrating organs with which the doctor is armed. From the subtle penetration of rays, the recording of heart or brain "waves," the fascinating graphics of abyssal operation, to the more direct search for a "cryptogenetic" disease through an exploration conducted using scopic equipment, that bring light in the caves of eternal bodily darkness, a desired rape is perpetrated, whose technique is speleological. Jumps, siphons, hoses, underground torrents, concretions and stones, stalactites of the inner caves, are finally seen, photographed, affected by "exploratory" laparotomies, this exhibitory game of "hide and seek" finding in the alter ego the complicity of a subject who examines, explores, inspects, palpates, and strikes (Maurel 1973).

Describing her pain as a continuous background to which sudden violent paroxysms were regularly added, Mrs. B. stating that she had just had a "crisis," solicited, as she had barely arrived, extra "serious examinations." Her judicious and appropriate use of medical discourse whose sometimes hermetic vocabulary seemed to have no secrets was striking. She expressed a great amazement, likely caused by the impression of a strange but familiar confrontation—in the sense of unheimliche—with a caricatured duplicate of the doctor.

Though necessary, the medical vocabulary was however powerless to fully express what Mrs. B. felt. Invited indeed, the day after her arrival, to clarify the exact nature of her pain, she repeatedly punctuated her speech with a rumbling, between belching and ventriloquism, and added every time, referring to a real language of the organs only able to represent them, "my pain is that." Besides speaking very extensively of her organs, Mrs. B. also seemed therefore to hear them and to make them talk, double eloquence in which we recognize the formation process of hypochondriac speech. In this connection, if the word *organon* meant tool or instrument in Greek before being applied to the systems of the body, note that it also was the name of the set of treaties that Aristotle devoted to logic, and that Thucydides more commonly used its plural, mainly in the sense of "forms of language," of "stylistic features (Bailly 1950, p.1396)." Hypochondria is therefore doubly organic: it is an "organ neurosis," but also a specific form and style of speech.

Mrs. B. was very quickly called "the Lady with the noise" by the care team, and in fact she caught their attention, as by a displacement, more because of the strangeness of this sound than because of the pain that it referred to. Very primitive way to attract attention? Possible regression of the relational mode to a "digestive voice" close to the wailing of the child? Informative value of these repeated noises which often suggested the swallowing of air, immediately expired? Obsessing manifestation perhaps comparable to a tic and referring of course, as noted by K. Abraham (Abraham 1966, p.133), to an anal-sadistic origin? Torture and suffering of a body in infinite gestation of an inarticulable Word? Many hypotheses can be put forward, inseparable from the form of psychic economy of the subject; their common point however seems to reside in the fact that they belong to a shared problem concerning the question of elusiveness and that of ineffability. In all cases, for our part, and in the absence of any positive report—except for "some originality" very frequently underlined—we apparently have to refer to the hypochondriac register to try to understand the present case, a sort of riddle, of Mrs. B. In the single and short interview that we could have with her, as she had refused to meet us the previous days, the total inability to discuss any other topic than this "disease" indicated, as in hypochondria, the way her psychic space was totally filled by its representation. Speaking with a remarkable prolixity, between two "hiccups," of the body which made her suffer, she never talked about her body as a whole and gave us in fact a perfectly similar discourse in all respects to the one she gave to doctors. Her verbal expression was however what stroke us first and foremost. In the beginning, there were just words, with no real syntactic construction. The vocabulary was conventional, the voice was flat, a sort of ventriloquism whose echo reached us, distant, the expression, somehow aloud, of a tremendously elusive soliloquy. She was not a subject who spoke to communicate, but someone who, at our request, barely threw the veil of silence on the numerous contradictions of her inner language, frightened at the noise that she made and remade and at the sense that it could receive when it was articulated out loud and especially at the address of another person. If we happened to respond or intervene, Mrs. B. ostensibly turned her head, evading the possible starting point of a true dialogue. The scientifico-hypochondriac considerations appear in their defense function, as an opening on a possibly significant theme, on an historical overview that would question the subject, invariably lead to a brief dumbstruck stop followed by the perpetual reference to past or future medical explorations. Under these very strange conditions, from her history and from what she was, in a prodigious tour de force, Mrs. B. had managed, with us as with the whole team, not to speak since her admission. Mrs. B. left us, very frustrated, with our countless questions and, deeply dissatisfied. Our lack appears, but isn't this precisely what she questioned?

4.2 Finding Complaint Invariants and Naming the Unnamable

In an attempt to summarize and synthesize them to highlight their main features, we can notice that the negative reports presented here, despite the extreme diversity of clinical contexts, reveal interesting invariants in somatic complaint with no detectable organic substrate; the constant conjunction of those invariants enables us to assert their undeniable unity as a discourse. The essential problem is therefore hypochondria in words that different constants articulate but also question. Isolating the main of them, we will strive to highlight how they are, each in turn, a partial aspect of the hypochondriac register considered as a model. Thus, we can distinguish:

(1) The regularly cranial and/or abdominal location of the symptoms which, in the absence of primary meaning and clear symbolism, conjures up the image, of typically anal character, of a hollow and closed cavity. Possible metaphor of a container whose dominant attributes could probably be found in the modalities of Interior and Depth, it precisely matches the central dimension of hypochondriac speech whose key words are "contain," "hold" and especially "stand" and then provide imagination with the opportunity to build a series of monsters, generally animated: fantasies of pregnancy for example, including the proximity of zoopathic characteristics expressed in medical parlance which can seemingly be observed in the case of Mrs. P.

(2) The relative euphemization of conflict in relation to the specific problems of the subjects which, often inseparable from an anomaly in the economy of affect, appears linked to a large alexithymic trend opposing, as in the psychosomatic patient, the verbalization of psychic pain (McDougall 1985, p.171). If in the two first cases conflict is somewhat superficially evoked and if it is indeed in the two others simply absent or set aside, the adult patients giving the impression, in some respects, to behave as nonverbal children at the mercy of others for the interpretation of their own mental states. In the interview situation, the concept of projective identification is this enlightening perspective which turns the interlocutor into a container to collect now what these past children have painfully learnt, i.e., that psychic survival depends on the ability to totally extinguish impulse.

(3) The permanent and heavy presence of depression, always at minimum, which, variously pervasive in each case, defensively seems to hide in their unequal importance internalized paranoid anxieties. If, as we have seen, a continuity of structure could effectively be identified between depression and hypochondria, guessed by the ancients under the unique term of neurasthenia, we can undoubtedly think that, in its mainly somatic form, the first is for the second a formidable auto-erotic counter-investment defense protecting the patient against a possible psychotic decompensation and a real suicidal danger during critical phases approaching more frankly the melancholic register (case of Mrs. C).

(4) The apparent and impressive "basal phantasmal inhibition" as evidenced by the discourse of all these patients. Manifested above all by a tireless repetition and the total lack of diversification, it invariably gives the impression of a "vacuum" or a "blank" in word assemblies where unexpected elements remain absent. The striking features here are the monoideism and mental poverty, simplicity also of an endless repetition of only mundane events. Patients seem to "ignore" all the things that they cannot relate to reality and its over-investment is a boring hyperrealism of the Tangible and Objective. Rather than in neurotic lineage, it is clearly in the psychosomatic field that we seemingly have to place them, interpreting them as J. Mc Dougall when she presents actual neuroses as the crucible of the latter (McDougall 1985, p.171).

(5) The central and capital relation of complaint as it is expressed, almost as an unlimited and especially unstoppable mixed demand for both life and pain suppression, with the basal level classically named "basic fault" by Balint in the sense of primarily referring to a lack of adjustment between mother and child, it truly seems to define a very typical object relation.

> It is definitely a two-person relationship in which, however, only one of the partners matters; his wishes and needs are the only ones that count and must be attended to; the other partner, though felt to be immensely powerful, matters only in so far as he is willing to gratify the first partner's needs and desires or decides to frustrate them (Balint 1967, p.23).

Description that is in a very close relationship with the mother's ability or inability to perform her function of barrier against excitement, presented by J. Mc. Dougall as one of the reasons why

> the children will grow up… remaining out of touch with important sectors of their psychic reality (McDougall 1985, p.197),

so significantly encountered in many psychosomatic patients.

(6) The important and real excitement in the words and expressions which invariably characterize most of these patients describing their boring somatic picture and their often atypical pains. Weakness of introjection and omnipotence of incorporation thus undoubtedly characterize a notable libidinal investment into the function of spoken language. What should be added is that this "phonatory auto-filling (Abraham and Torok 1978, pp.208–212)," for

which the other person is used as a mirror, obviously reminds of the specific status of word in hypochondria. Through repeated descriptions, an ill person creates a real trompe-l'oeil on the invisibility of his wounds: he attracts the attention of a look when only his text, in fact, monopolizes him. When he seems to invest his words as organs, he perhaps organizes them in his discourse, as being his real pains, similar on this point to the hypochondriac and at the same time very close to a manic position.

Therefore, the recourse to hypochondria primarily invites to question and study the register in which it fits. The reported proximity of the field of mood disorders ("depression") and its kinship not less underlined with the psychosomatic sphere ("nonelaboration") enable to use interconnected various figures and terms.

A point atop all cases however retains us a little, which is primarily economic. It is actually with some reasons that if, from eclectic issues, all of the subjects uniformly encountered, as no name could be given to the "disease" mentioned, expressed their situation and experience around a part of their anatomy in what we can call the true substitute for a "relationship of/to the unknown (Rosolato 1978, p.228)," and fanatically believed that they could find in medicine and caregivers what they saw as their salvation. It should be noted however that, very often, their loss also was as contained in this rush. Unlimited quest for diagnosis and accusation of persecution indeed almost ceaselessly alternated, as well as long incantations to medical victories and appropriation of this verbal power, in a unique entanglement, at the level of therapeutic action, of good and evil, of omnipotence and helplessness. How can medical discourse generate such a paradoxical approach? Perhaps, like hypochondriacs, the patients which we are dealing with, somehow spot in it a way to understand the body in its entirety, which they frantically hope. And, all things considered, they are not wrong to think that on the horizon of the art here practiced, there is a biological body that, once evil will be eradicated, could be anonymous, devoid of any mark or secret, silent and full, liberated from hassle and history, pure health. What to say then but that, always keeping the crazy hope to substitute the biological body to the necessarily marked and erogenous one, excluding death and time, thanks to the hope continuously offered by medicine, the complaining subjects think they can try, in a real hocus-pocus, to annihilate and destroy this unspeakable that they believe they convey? The illusion of a body that might be protected from castration, i.e., from evil and pain, from desire, away from death, is especially important for them, protected from castration which seems to be continually expressed in the real body through the constantly renewed evocation of cruel pains. From there, their hopes dissociate into two major trends. From the reference to the body of totalitarian science and to the apparent protection from castration that this suggests, indeed comes the threat of persistent and very alienating intrusions: iatrogenic doctor, persecuting doctor then looks like the serious evidence that one cannot really adhere to such a speech for long without reaping its painful feedback. Of course, multiple tricks are possible: a doctor reduced to no power and no knowledge, solution that reduces risks and hopes; the partial or total appropriation of the vocabulary of the medical profession can also be a radical bias, but it requires a difficult learning and provides little relief. Everything happens as if, similarly to hypochondria, a single question endlessly arose, desperately challenging the physician: "Un-mark my body, but, above all, do not put your mark on it. Name my unspeakable, but above all do not leave your name on it." Demand in which we can recognize one of the actual formulations of the denial of castration by fetishization of the body.

Chapter 5
From Biological Body to Metaphorical Body

Abstract On the one hand, we expound a criticism of the concept of Actuality that induces us to reject the Freudian bi-dimensional evolutionist model. More specifically, we explain how the Freudian etiology that attributes actual neurosis to the stasis of ego-libido conceals ambiguities and contradictions. On the other hand, we demonstrate that, as clinical observation reveals a continuity between hypochondria, sleep, and soma, the fact that biological and psychoanalytical approaches are mutually exclusive constitutes a stumbling block. We explain how anasemia enables us to go beyond this obstacle and why we must focus on the meaning of the hypochondriac's denial of medical power.

5.1 Register of Actuality

If the register of hypochondria as a possible reading mode for the exposed cases prompts to interrogate its nature and at the same time induces to question the register of ACTUALITY that it belongs to, we must first of all probably clarify what Freud said about it. The difficulty and ambiguity of such a reminder, however, must be reported, as an effect and even a reflection of the contradictions and flaws inherent in his conception of actual neuroses, conception linked to a theory which, proposing among other functions to consider and develop the important issue of somatizations, presents a two-dimension model based on the opposition of neurotic and actual. Described by M. Sami-Ali as bi-dimensional, it consists in admitting that, in contrast to psychoneurotic symptoms that invariably refer to repression, to the failure of repression and to the return of the repressed, possibly through somatic expression, the symptoms of actual neuroses (hypochondria, anxiety neurosis, neurasthenia) result, with no mediation, of possible disturbances of the sexual metabolism whose decrease or unbridled increase they reflect, with no signification. Freud said it very variously evoking them in the form of

> intracranial pressure, sensations of pain, a state of irritation in an organ, weakening or inhibition of a function (Freud 1916–1917, p.387)

M. Derzelle, *Towards a Psychosomatic Conception of Hypochondria*, 59
DOI: 10.1007/978-3-319-03053-1_5,
© Springer International Publishing Switzerland 2014

that are meaningless symptoms. More exactly, unlike the primary meaning of psychoneurotic symptoms, they may only have a secondary meaning, acquired after the fact, that does not trigger the process of symptomatic formation, and this keeps them away from any symbolism of causal type. Even if Graves' disease, invoked by Freud himself in support of his remarks, may mean a guilt being atone, it is nonetheless true that, from the point of view of causation, it is due to

> toxins which are not introduced into the body from outside but originate in the subject's own metabolism (Freud 1916–1917, p.388).

Guilt is then an attempt to rationalize a state of hormonal disorder whose true etiology is in another sphere. Therefore, actual symptoms are, for Freud, entirely physical.

> They are not only manifested in the body (as are hysterical symptoms, for instance, as well), but they are also themselves entirely somatic processes, in the generating of which all the complicated mental mechanisms we have come to know are absent (Freud 1916–1917, p.387).

And if, despite this fact, they are within the Freudian corpus, it is thanks to the energy concept of libido which brings together actual and neurotic in the sexual function which is not a,

> purely psychical thing any more than it is a somatic one (Freud 1916–1917, p.388).

The evocation of these indications however allows to point out that if the psychosomatic disorders are quite conceivable from the analytical perspective because of their compliance with the described neuroses as referring to actuality, the allocation, maintained by Freud throughout his life, of the original cause of these to the disorders of actual sexual life appears, on the other hand little appropriate in the light of current psychoanalytic thought.

The question arises then about how to articulate actual and neurotic, and about what is indeed specific in the register of actuality, related first of all by Freud to actualized sexual practices, justifying that it could be qualified so. In fact, if we consider terminology, the word "actual" has a chronological meaning, neuroses designed as actual primarily resulting from disorders of the sexuality lived currently: "actual", on this point, only equals "contemporary". You might also think that by some sort of contiguity, "actual" in this context means something close to "manifest" in the sense that Freud frequently opposed it to the term "latent". Strictly asemic because of their total corporeality, actual neuroses do indeed hide no cryptic content needing an anamnestic investigation to be appreciated. Finally "actual", with a real semantic ambiguity, refers to the Act in a pluralist way. In this regard, J. Laplanche and J. B. Pontalis noted moreover that the verb *Agieren* (translated by acting out, turning into Act)

> has an ambiguity which is in Freud's thought itself: he confuses what, in transference, is actualization and what resorts to driving action, which is not necessarily implied by transference (Laplanche and Pontalis 1967, p.240).

Similarly, in the field of actual neuroses, a reference to driving action is involved, that Freud described as "inadequate" or even "diverted" (Freud 1973b, p.33). More importantly, in a quite basal way, the actual symptom here is equivalent to the action and discharge which constitute the normal coitus (Freud 1973b, p.35). What matters here is indeed sexual intercourse: actual neuroses would so be, strictly speaking, disorders of sexuality as an act, that this is expressed, with no distinction, by an inadequate discharge of drive or an equivalent that is nonexplicitly driving the action. From these different interpretations, ranging beyond contradictions, emerges the essential idea of a body sex-endowed before even being a sexual body, which clearly refers to the register of actuality as a necessary and fundamental anchor. Archaicity and actuality both refer to the sex-endowed body, while the neurotic level, more elaborate and more psychological, refers to the symbolic body, in a gradation that is much more topical than chronological. Archaic zones which are "not neurotized", mysterious reflections of the biological body, can very well be anchored within subjects with neurotic traits. This coexistence must be highlighted as, besides it applies to the mentioned cases, it enables to think the register of actuality and the one of neurosis as synchronic more than diachronic concepts.

5.2 Freud and Hypochondria: "Secondary" Narcissism

The various notations that Freud devoted in particular to the very point of hypo-chondria, also have, by many sides, these imperfections and contradictions already identified in his theory about the context of actual neuroses. The first difficulty lies in that, throughout his reflection, the classic distinction between major or psychotic hypochondria and minor or neurotic hypochondria does never retain his attention, joining in this a clinical tradition for which, even when it is "simple" and "minor", hypochondria thought as a single actual neurosis is always somewhat seen as "vesanic". This very important and heavy ambiguity is visible, and not without effects, in the three citations selected here to show how Freud deals with the subject and taken from his study of the Schreber case (1911), from *On Narcissism: an Introduction.* (1914) and from *Introductory Lectures on Psycho-Analysis* (1916)

- In the earlier of these writings, we see Freud rally, concerning Psychiatry, the nineteenth century way of thinking which tends to emphasize, noting its frequency, the real and often meaningful coincidence of chronic delusion with the disease named hypochondria.

  I must not omit to remark at this point that I shall not consider any theory of paranoia trustworthy unless it also covers the hypochondriacal symptoms by which this disorder is almost invariably accompanied. It seems to me that hypochondria stands in the same relation to paranoia as anxiety neurosis does to hysteria (Freud 1911, pp. 56–57).

This had already been noted by Morel who stated that delusions of persecution were ultimately only a transformation of hypochondria. And Magnan, considering the "chronic delusion" during its so-called "incubation" phase, writes the same way:

At this stage of the disease, it really looks like hypochondria (Magnan and Sérieux 1890, p.43).

In his "psychoanalytic study of a case of paranoia", it is however the interesting question of the instance of hypochondria in it that Freud, resorting to analogy, asks, without answering it in precise terms. Yet we can see him expose some parts of his theory, pointing in his remarks, among other elements, the famous "detachment of libido":

the liberated libido becomes attached to the ego, and is used for the aggrandizement of the ego (Freud 1911, p.72).

But this "fixation at the stage of narcissism" is only mentioned to report, in fact, the delusions of grandeur, while its affinity with hypochondria is, in some way, not really developed.

- *To introduce Narcissism* more directly addresses the topic and deserves a much closer analysis. This work, one of the tipping points of Freud's theoretical progress, demonstrates as a priority that

    distinguishing a sexual libido from a nonsexual energy of the ego-instincts (Frued 1914, p.76)

    is possible, that this distinction

    corresponds to the common popular distinction between hunger and love (Freud 1914, p.78)

and can no doubt also help us find, for hypochondria, a better approach of the modalities of orality. The direct study of narcissism yet faces "difficulties" here described as "special," and, all in all, its only "access road" remains the "analysis of paraphrenias", i.e., for Freud, as usual, dementia praecox or schizophrenia always accompanied by paranoia. There are however "some other ways", which "remain open" for exploration, and that Freud prefers to investigate. Among them, banal but unique, we can first distinguish all diseases in their organic dimension: the patient "withdraws his libido investment on his ego", which results in "the well-known selfishness of the patient".

Then, in the same way, totally similar phenomena occur in sleep,

a narcissistic withdrawal of the positions of the libido on to the subject's own self.

    Then and finally comes hypochondria: The hypochondriac withdraws both interest and libido... from the objects of the external world and concentrates both of them upon the organ that is engaging his attention (Freud 1914, p.83).

No doubt we still need to insist on the adjacency, already mentioned, of the soma-sleep-hypochondria continuum whose obvious link here seems to arise at first from the structure of the text itself, confirmed and even "aggravated" by the then expressed conjecture:

hypochondria must be right, organic changes must be present in it (Freud 1914, p.83).

The genital organ, when it is excited, is "the model of a painfully sensitive organ;" specifically, erogeneity can be considered as "a general characteristic of all organs" (Freud 1914, p.84). Changes in the investment of libido in the ego would therefore correspond to alterations in the erogeneity of organs, and when he implies that they are material, the author suggests the true character of these changes, giving them a place in the great concert of actual neuroses. But hypochondria is distinguished, in fact, from the other neuroses of this type as anxiety neurosis and neurasthenia because it depends, very differently and on the contrary, on libido taking the subject's ego as its object.

hypochondriacal anxiety is the counterpart, as coming from ego-libido, to neurotic anxiety (Freud 1914, p.84);

This would involve, by extrapolation of and by reference to the theory of actual neuroses, that it would result in fact, without any mediation whatsoever, of the outright transformation of the ego-libido attached to an organ, into anxiety. Freud does not formulate this proposal, but it seems that he suggests it by the fact that he classifies hypochondria among actual neuroses.

Going further, Freud then concentrates on considering the modalities of paraphrenias:

The libido that is liberated by frustration does not remain attached to objects in phantasy, but withdraws on to the ego (Freud 1914, p.86),

"delusions of grandeur" being nothing less, in these conditions, that an attempt of inner development, of "mastery of this mass of libido", strictly speaking fantasy without an object or, more accurately, to be truthful, with no other possible object than only narcissistic. Hence the failure, and

Perhaps it is only when the megalomania fails that the damming-up of the ego becomes pathogenic

Then

the hypochondria of paraphrenia... homologous to the anxiety of transference neuroses (Freud 1914, p.86),

would emerge from this failure.

If this formulation gives a solution to the problem raised but unsolved concerning the affliction of President Schreber, it however appears to hardly agree with the Freudian conceptions exposed above, which consider hypochondria as an actual neurosis (Freud 1914, p.84). But perhaps we should imagine that the facts presented in theoretical scope are only valid in the case of the psychotic form? We have already said it: in his texts, Freud never definitely refers to a splitting of this single affliction that would allow the study of two different forms of hypochondria. He always calls it "neurosis", but we believe that we can understand "psychosis", since the large group of "narcissistic neuroses" means in fact, on the nosographic level, the major psychoses identified as chronic.

- Finally if we seek some clarification in *Introduction to psychoanalysis*, we mainly find a repetition of the arguments already developed in the work previously analyzed (Freud 1916–1917, p.419–421). Again in fact, Freud compares hypochondria, presented in his remarks as the logical continuation of a narcissistic withdrawal of libido, to illness. Detached from objects under the influence of a "determined, very energetic process", libido

  that has become narcissistic cannot find its way back to objects, and this interference with the libido's mobility certainly becomes pathogenic as It seems that an accumulation of narcissistic libido beyond a certain amount is not tolerated (Freud 1916–1917, p.421).

In fact, what we can find here is the notion of "stasis of the libido of the ego," but this time Freud no longer mentions the failure of the attempt of a pseudo-fantasmatic elaboration whose theme is organized by the inflation of the ego. This text is however, as the previous two, filled with the thorns of ambiguity. Thus, when he tries to complete the theory of actual neuroses, Freud recalls that hypochondria falls within this category whose symptomatology is said to have "no meaning", and yet he seeks and finds, despite this insistence, "a direction for the understanding of hypochondria".

This contradiction can be kept, in which we can find the guideline of a hermeneutic approach. But its ambiguities and difficulties complicate the study of this theory called "narcissistic". J. Lacan also very aptly pointed it, by writing:

The very notion of narcissistic attachment... remains very insufficient, as evidenced by the confusion of ongoing discussions on... the very economic value of symptoms that most securely found the theory of narcissism (symptoms of depersonalization, hypochondriacal ideas): are these phenomena libidinal overinvestment or disinvestment? On this point opinions differ completely (Lacan 1932, p.333); and further: narcissism... is considered, in the economy of psychoanalytic doctrine, as a *terra incognita;* the means of investigation resulting from the study of neuroses has identified its borders, but its interior remains mythical and unknown (Lacan 1932, p.334).

5.3 Somatic Complaint, Suffering of an Insomniac Body

Considering Freud's exact contribution, despite the contradictions inherent in his theory, to the study of hypochondria, it seems that three main points emerge, which are at the core of the Freudian contribution:

(1) We can first notice how late Freud really addressed this issue only devoting a short time (1911–1916) to it, while it is paradoxically, in the most intimate proximity with the first clinical entity isolated by him as a topical syndrome (1895). It should probably therefore primarily be proposed, more than as a well-differentiated complex, as a modality of ACTUALITY, an already built theoretical corpus in which it later appears (1914) whose difficulty Freud has never ceased to see and say when he found it at all the turns of his pathway.

(2) It is also important to point the unity of hypochondria, for Freud, no distinction being made between the one that frankly turns to delusion and the less tragic psychoneurotic one, which affects many clinical cases. Despite the current label of actual neurosis that serves as header, everything allows to think that Freud thought that it was closer to chronic psychosis than to neuroses. For him, it might be the heart and core of paraphrenia, while the similar diseases, going hand in hand, are referred to as "transference neuroses." Its very close ties to the key concept of "libido of the ego" and its really authentic relationship to the theory known as "narcissistic" still keep it further away from these last two.

(3) We can finally note the case of exception, problematic to think, that hypochondria consists in, as it has a double status both parts of which must be maintained. As an actual neurosis, it always temporally precedes the psychoneurotic clinical expression, it indeed seems to constitute a key background in the all narcissistic disorders that are the paraphrenic syndromes and, among these, paranoia. Freud did not attempt to develop a logical theoretical system, but his hypotheses are worth clinical interest as they, from a metapsychological perspective, locate sleep and disease as of organic nature in close proximity to hypochondria.

This continuity, already mentioned, between hypochondria, sleep, and soma is indeed the point that we will consider, in that it seems to allow us to clearly think from a fantasmatic point of view the metaphorized "somatic" fact that medicine can think, and thereby also to designify, by considering how concepts relate to one another, what the somatic complainant expresses of an issue entirely centered on regression and narcissism. The metapsychological theoretical perspective is an inherently transgressive epistemology, which intrinsically confers all its prerogatives to it, and it indeed enables us to reconsider the scientific data, not to avoid them but to obtain the drive motion from them, by gradually pushing each conceptual resistance backwards and making them fall. As properly said, thus, by P. Fedida:

> Whether we are to define drive as a boundary concept or its doctrine as a mythology, whether we are to think the hypochondriacal organ on the model of a painfully sensitive organ, modified in a certain way without yet being sick in the usual sense, whether we finally are (but examples are not restrictive here) to call a definition of physical pain in terms of melancholy: every time, we think scientifically unthinkable ideas from a fantasmatic point of view (Fedida 1978a, p.625).

Then, there is no possible junction between a biological theory of the soma and the psychoanalytic theory, each science becoming necessarily "false" when thought rises to the level of fantasy. And this "falsity", which can be considered heuristic implies that the metapsychological concept should in fact designifiy established content, in the process that N. Abraham called "anasemia" when he showed how, once de-signified, the word "somatic" obliges to operate the same activity on the word "psychical" to which it is linked (Abraham and Torok 1978, pp.208–212). "Anasemia", he says, based on the finding of the true relationship known as somato-psychical that J. Laplanche and J. B. Pontalis try to identify by a comparison to "delegation" at the end of the article "psychic representative (Laplanche and Pontalis 1967, p.240),"

> anasemia here is found in the term somatic with the biological sense of the word, and the same can be said of organic in similar context. To speak of a relation of mission, it would be necessary to attribute to the emissary traits in common with the sender, on the one hand, and with the accrediting party on the other hand. Its mediating function should be that of communication through interpreters and would merely imply difference of language, not of nature, between the two poles of the relation. It is understood that, under these conditions, somatic can no longer mean "somatic" but something else, and that, similarly, psychic finds itself de-signified as well; only the representative, the mediator between the two poles x, seems to have preserved its meaning, inasmuch as it is a term known by comparison (Abraham and Torok 1978, pp.211).

In this perspective, the patient's somatic complaints without any patent organic substrate can be heard speaking of something different from real somatic content in the current substantial and causal sense, even if the latter nevertheless appears to be "used" for certain purposes. This new listening where the "Somatic" responds to the triple criterion of a topical function, but also of an economics and a dynamics promotes it thus first and foremost to metaphorically convey, in words, without being said as such, what is in fact actually the work of instinctual life. But we must add that this transformation, which can be done only in the condition of a relevant de-signification, is made possible by the indications that Freud gave on a "mythical" definition of the word "somatic" through the fundamentally narcissistic sleep-dream relationship where the oneiric body gives us access to a specific somatic truth (Freud 1915[1917]a, p.223).

> We mean that the only possible understanding of the Somatic is this metapsychology of sleep in such a way that no psychology of dreams can exist… Dream is for the body its own myth and the only possible place—that is analytical—of its interpretation (Fedida 1977b, p.54).

If, from a strict metapsychological point of view, dream is preeminently a somatic theory, the close proximity between it and hypochondria, as we have underlined it above, can then be fruitful for our subject. When we confront them and make them interact in their essential complementarity, it seems in fact that the hypochondriac, very privileged theorist of the "somatic fact" as "de-signified", suffers from a sleepless body. The explanation of this idea is that it induces to consider what relates and differentiates the areas of dream and hypochondria. Their contiguity emerges in the fact that they involve, in a unique and similar way, the basal narcissistic withdrawal which characterizes investment in the Somatic (Freud 1914, p.83) and allows Freud to credit dream with remarkable and unquestionable diagnostic powers:

The diagnostic capacity of dreams—a phenomenon which is generally acknowledged but regarded puzzling—becomes equally comprehensible, too. In dreams, incipient physical disease is often detected earlier and more clearly than in waking life, and all the current bodily sensations assume gigantic proportions. And this magnification is hypochondriacal in character, it is conditional upon the withdrawal of all psychical cathexes from the external world back on to the ego, and it makes possible early recognition of bodily changes which would still for a time have remained unobserved (Freud 1915[1917]a, p.223).

But hypochondria is also a close companion of insomnia in that, on two specific points, it really deviates and differs from dream, as noted by P. Fedida when he developed elements of this rich but delicate path (Fedida 1977b, pp.51–65):

(1) Dream and hypochondria are opposed without compromise on what might be called a mourning of oneself. If, by recourse to hallucination, dream is, of a possible death that sleep simulates, a resolution, hypochondria however refuses death and looks after the affected organ as "transparency of oneself" restlessly speaking the pain in words. This last is thereby placed in a relationship of choice toward mourning, average position between completed mourning and the franc refusal of this process, impossibility—we must point it—characteristic of the melancholic whose ego phantasmatically "swallows" the object to which he was attached by an often very ambivalent link. An equivalence between hypochondria and melancholia must also be considered and outlined: incorporation is triumphant, but introjection is almost nonexistent.

(2) Dream and hypochondria are still very radically opposed on the last object of their investments. If the work of dream restlessly reveals a permanent path opening on the unconscious, in the hypochondriac, on the contrary, the investment of the word that hallucinates the organ warns that that of the "thing" is sorely lacking. Because, as Freud rightly says:

It is very noteworthy how little the dream-work keeps to word-presentation, it is always ready to exchange one word for another till it finds the expression which is most handy for plastic representation (Freud 1915[1917]a, p.228).

The substitution of images to thoughts is therefore the result of a work aimed at reducing words representations to thing representations

as if, in general, the process were dominated by considerations of representability (Freud 1915[1917]a, p.227).

In hypochondria, this communication is no more effective as if, become a prey to insomnia, the subject seemed deprived of any ability to dream, that is, in fact, to find

in the representations of things a hallucinatory satisfaction of desire that only the somatic allows in sleep (Fedida 1977b, p.60).

These considerations show a confirmation of the proposed hypothesis, the relationship of somatic complaint with dream giving the impression to be similar to the one perversion, especially when it is fetishization, apparently has with sexual infantile theories (Freud 1908, pp.205–226). Like these, it is indeed as the conclusion, in a certain way, of primary processes, that oneiric fact holds a part of truth called "somatic", while complaint and perversion mark a lack of connection to the unconscious. The analogy can be pursued with the relationship to mourning. If in the first case, mourning of the object, "accepted" as lost, is made, freeing investment that can then be transferred onto other objects (desire to know, dream), in the second case, refusing the loss, complaint, and perversion hallucinate the ABSENT, that then plays an important part.

Somatic complaint with no organic substrate: what we have here is a grief work that has not yet been done.

> The absent is then the hatred object of love. Thought can, thus, find itself empty for thinking it too much. Emptiness whose inside is unoccupied because waiting is suspended when anxiety is removed. White pain of the absent (Fedida 1978b, p.7).

5.4 From Medicalized Body to Thought Body

How can the biological body become a psychological body? How can nonelaborated and nonpsychized areas become elements of dream or thought? That is *the* question that we have never ceased to identify and which, very central on the theoretical level, is not without effect on the clinical approach. J. B. Pontalis and J. Mc Dougall seem here to have the capacity to talk about these two aspects.

> The path which starts from the imageless fragmentary primary body which is unrepresentable for the psyche, to lead to the unified erogenous body which is a subject of fantasies and an object of symbolization, is sometimes crisscrossed, suddenly cut-off, full of confusing traces. For whom desperately attempts to follow the tracks of this pathway in the tortuous maze of an analysis, the emotional current, as a privileged connection between soma and psyche, is offered as a guide through its thousand disguises. But what happens when this vivid torrent, searching scenes, fantasies, words, to contain and ballast its flow, finds no access to psychic representation? Emotional currents can either be triggered by the instinctual pulsation or mobilized by the continuous impact of the external world, they endlessly gush from the depths of every being. What route do they take? (McDougall 1982, p.152)

> Between dream and pain, it is also what appears to me as the field of analytic experience, in its permanent swing between what can be said—displaced, censored, denied—but said, or which can be represented—disguised, truncated, misleading—but expressed, and what, to be heard, needs to be either silent or yelling: sometimes the unspoken is not simply the erasure of what would have been said elsewhere or before. At one pole, there is dream, prototype of the formations of the unconscious, where the contradictory wishes of childhood can both be accomplished and deciphered; dream: object of anxiety and delight, of nostalgia and... analysis. At the other pole, there is pain, which blurs the boundaries between body and psyche, conscious and unconscious, me and the other, outside and inside; pain: surely at the limits of analysis but in the, absent, very center, of our word, masked gap that the ordeal of grief and madness may still reopen (Pontalis 1977, p.8).

Part III
Thinking Hypochondria

Introduction

Abstract First, clinical observation reveals that hypochondria is above all a belief, which relates it to the concept of projection. Then, the cruciality of the concepts of impasse and transference is demonstrated. These reflections lead us to new problematics on the required theoretical model and to new concepts that will ensure a rigorous and fruitful study of hypochondria.

Voluntarily focused on four clinical cases, our first research perspective, making full use of the Freudian system, does indeed appear of limited interest as if it operated aporetically. If hypochondria is to be defined in continuity with the Somatic as well as with the oneiric process, it is clear that this common 'x' linked to narcissism remains an enigma and a lacuna in the Freudian model: the two aspects of the same aporia, both referring to a single question on the body as belonging to the imaginary level and the real level, consist in the theoretical status of Somatic that obliges to conceive everything as psychic apparatus on the one hand, and in the never developed articulation between dream and the projective process on the other hand. And we must add, in order to elaborate a conceptualization intended to express this dual dimension as a global system absorbing health and disease in a continuum and enabling to think hypochondria, that we can find in Freud a meaningful intuition in the heart of the field of normality: it was, belatedly, in 1917, normal prototype of morbid phenomena, dream, considered as a projection.

> A dream tells us that something was going on which tended to interrupt sleep, and it enables us to understand in what way it was possible to fend off this interruption. The final outcome is that the sleeper has dreamt and is able to go on sleeping; the internal demand which was striving to occupy him has been replaced by an external experience whose demand has been disposed of. A dream is, therefore, among other things, a projection, an externalization of an internal process (Freud 1915[1917]a).

Far from having here a defensive function, projection is a possibility for the subject to create, outside of him, a world that is him and that he turns it into his object: radical misconception of a body turned into a world, ignorance of the subject thinking that he is another, it is a synonym of imagination with the meaning of a mode of thinking constantly turning the subject into objects and whose nocturnal dream is only a modality.

What is at stake in this contribution is important. First it allows to pose the problem of projection in its entirety, this problem whose promised analysis never came (Freud 1911; 1912–1913; 1915[1917]a) and which prevented the elaboration of a theory of the body, it allows to find new focus points for a possible research intended to remold concepts in order to really understand hypochondria. Because if imagination is nothing but dream and its equivalents when we are awake, this finding offers an interpretation framework, diverting from symptoms i.e., the Intrapsychic to relational life i.e., the Interpsychical pointing hypochondria as an expression of what is only a variant of dream, in conditions that are different from sleep. This re-orientation, in the form of a hypothesis, can be done by following a triple reference that allows a framing of the issue and of its situation but also has the immense advantage of linking aspects that are necessarily excluded by an energetic conception. The following directions, notes and related cases that exceed the Freudian metapsychology emerge from the questioned concrete clinical observations:

(1) From the point of view of affect, hypochondria seems to constitute a form of belief.
(2) Within the relationship as it is initiated in a medical clinical situation, the concept of impasse seems to articulate several plans ranging from complaint to the system itself.
(3) From the point of view of transference, hypochondria might be interpreted as an attempt to perhaps elaborate a relational impasse situation, on the background of an early relationship of paradoxical type.

Let us explain these points more precisely.

1. From the point of view of affect first, something is obvious. If what we mean by hypochondria is not a condition, subjective translation within a closed system of a specific quantity of instinctual energy as it is postulated in an economic theory, but rather a highly personalized internal reaction associated with a relational situation and that has a place in the story of the subject, it is constantly clear, that, in the middle of numerous negatives affects always repeating the same sequence where trust and mistrust constantly alternate, the major feature of the hypochondriac is a hard, firm and unshakeable belief. Belief in a body mysteriously affected, ill in spite of everything, in spite of doctors also, and that cannot change even when faced with obvious facts. Belief in a body affected "in advance" that the confrontation with a body of knowledge, in the absence of any term used as a third instance, always leaves unshaken afterwards. The link to psychosis is obviously necessary, as well as to the forms delusional experience of the body, since reality is bracketed here: the visible

and knowable reality is held aside, putting reality testing out of the game while knowledge on reality is maintained in the form of "consultation." Hypochondria is therefore a denial process which both cancels and accepts, in the same movement, a knowledge on reality where the body, occurrence of a limited delusion, played the role of a fundamentally impossible object. Ill, the hypochondriac uses the other person, the doctor, in the quest for a probable future healing. Considered healthy, he maintains this need, in the quest for the naming of a possible illness. In either case, as a kind of link to the other, what prevails is the belief in what you can name the dreamlike value of words expressing complaint: the condition of organs depends on their saying, likely to induce change in the other person. Thus we can find the answer, in terms of belief, to our first question: dream equivalent in daytime life, like fantasy, game, illusion, and delusion, hypochondria seems to be a variant of projection (Sami-Ali 1982).

2. In the relationship as it is initiated in a medical clinical situation, more than ambivalence, which has descriptive value and can be found in the symptoms, what we speak about is a situation of impasse, as the belief in body affection includes a relationship to the other person on which the complaint depends. Far from consisting in the coexistence within the same subject of two opposing motions or in a permanent co-occurrence of opposite qualities within the same object, hypochondria as such is indeed in the form of a relational configuration: what happens to the body is constantly conveyed by a relationship with the Medical that, far from constituting an external element is primarily at the heart of physical suffering. In this situation, the concept of impasse, which expresses a figure whose logical structure is essentially that of a contradiction, closing all the exits, close to the unthinkable as well as to the nonelaborable of the psychotic conflict, enables to designate, as well as a mode of operation, an untenable situation: as objective examination does not stop complaint, health and disease seem to be equivalents within an endless relationship of absolute dependence that both gives and withdraws being. This concept of impasse concerns at least three levels:

– It first means the objective impasse linked to the medical situation itself which, to address the issue focusing on complaint in its function of a call for a resolution (Clavreul 1978, p.151), conceals that it depends on a manner to apprehend the other person as provided with influence. Then hypochondria loses all its intersubjective dimension, this exemplary coalescence between two characters tied around a drama and around the search for a fluctuating object: as negative responses never confirm, for the hypochondriac, the absence of disease, his request is reversed, once it is denied, he wants to be sick rather than to be healed. The impossibility of relief, generated by affirmative as well as negative answers, reveals the terms of a similarly impossible choice: the requirement of a cure arises concurrently with a belief of incurability, the hope for a naming with a strategy of evasivity.

– It expresses the resulting therapeutic impasse, clinical medicine addressing the symptoms while the problem in question happens first and foremost in a relationship. This shows how a second impasse is added to the first one, demonstrating what we suspected, i.e., that the other person can have control on the body and that suffering reflects this power; this impasse refers to the physician as unable to heal and not wanting to heal, trying to crush you. The impasse purely related to the medical system only feeds a purpose: asking not be healed in order to live, chronically maintaining the question, constituting the doctor as a double just as mysterious as the evil that takes you. An impossible approach responds to the impossible. Paradox of a double impossibility: of repair and separation. For the alteration which seems in question might be an unrepresentable otherness whose realization could be fatal...

– It finally stresses the theoretical impasse that is inseparable from this double impasse which results from the Freudian theory, instinctual theory of a complete object, where pathology is intrapsychic. But if we stay on a strictly descriptive level naming symptoms and operation modes, hypochondria remains a prevented thought associated with a blocked situation. The way out of the impasse, both theoretical and clinical, requires another system of thought and should probably begin with its acknowledgment in order to clear the terms of its formulation. This means that the absolute primacy of relationship must be postulated as a first requirement, so as to ask the questions pertaining to the impasse and in order to consider what type of relationship they are a repetition of. To the purely economic notion of a libido stasis within a closed system, a new dimension will be substituted: that of an unconscious as relationship to the other person, on which the escape from confinement depends.

3. From the point of view of transference, it seems that the objective impasse has to be read as the repetition of a subjective impasse on the relational level, projective attempt of a restoration of the relationship to the other person, on the model of childhood. This proposal, minimum framing of future development, feeds on a return to our four clinical cases intended to highlight all the internal as well as external combinable conditions underlying the problem, in these specific subjects and in a given time that is, in their story, a particular time. Here, we will make successive observations:

– Everything happens as if, a "life event" linked to absence or difference and always found in the observed cases, only revealed an earlier adapted state collapsing due to an intolerance to metabolize, in an operation mode to be specified, a distress or conflict situation generating an impasse situation. The equivalent of an identity disorder appears in cases I and IV when the other person disappears, the spouse in fact, by divorce or death (detail given to us by Mrs. B.), making real and symbolic equivalent. The same disorder exists in cases II and III when the other person exposes his or her otherness: the girl child reveals sexual difference (II) whereas the extent of the gap between the face of the wife and that of the mother repeatedly arises in Mr. C. (III) the insistent regret that "she" is not like "her." Difference and absence become an irreducible aspect of a condition which excludes these possibilities.

– The loss felt, in either case, is that of an all-powerful maternal figure, on which the subject depends in his identity by coincidence of to be and to have to. In the diverse forms of a tyrannical husband, forbidding studies, and all other projects (I), of an employer with a sadistic attitude and potentially highly conflicting orders (II), of a wife with which by splitting, the psyche of the patient is identified (III), of finally another person who utters the text whose mumbled echo constitutes the subject (IV), it is indeed still what Sami-Ali, in his theory, called the "body superego" (Sami-Ali 1987, p.66 note 1) which, through its evasion, is of the nature of the unthinkable because the subject's feeling of being depends on it, and seems to open up the breach in an operation mode where prohibition of being equates being. Death of the single object that is the unique subject: the absence of executioner is a harbinger of death. Unless you manage to think the unthinkable...

– Last striking finding made while proofreading the reported stories: that of an oscillation between hypochondria and allergic symptoms. Indeed, their medical history testifies to the common presence of those in childhood (Mrs. C.: eczema at the age of 4; Mrs. P.: childhood eczema and giant hives; M. G.: many episodes of sinusitis and allergic rhinitis; Mrs. B.: frequent asthma attacks through adolescence); but it is also probably worthwhile to point out that, in three cases out of four, somatic complaint seems to have established in the immediate aftermath of an allergic problem accompanying a loss: at each birth, Mrs. P. indicates the presence of eczema in the head and hands; Mr. C. clearly dates the quasi-permanence of rhinitis crises to his recent wedding; finally, Mrs. B. according to her file, was hospitalized immediately after her widowhood for an important "status asthmaticus" that she had not experienced for over thirty years! As if hypochondria absorbed allergy, in an affinity which must be thought...

This reorientation therefore helps a reformulation of the problem. Because if hypochondria is first and foremost a belief including in its cipher a relationship to the other person, in addition to the fact that it contradicts the notion of Actual conceived as purely physical symptoms, it means at the same time that we should consider as null and void any two-dimensional model that would introduce a radical break between two dimensions of the Somatic thought in relation to transference, positively as well as negatively. What is then involved is the definition of Psychic and Somatic, and the relations linking the former to the latter then need to be thought differently since the notion of propping is improper to identify what is posed as a clinical symptomatic variability. The three big questions which should be raised as problematics, questions within the Freudian system that can only be answered if we go beyond its limits, are therefore replaced with the following questions when the hypochondriac turns out to be a believer:

(1) What theoretical model can we use to think this object included in a relational pathology, admitting the contribution of Freudian metapsychology without being reduced to it?

(2) What basic concept(s) would allow to read hypochondria as a form of pathology which equally includes the operating mode of the concerned subjects and the situations that they might have had to face, conflicting situations that are elaborable or not?

(3) How finally could we think the variability of which hypochondria seems to be a deployment and how to conceive this proximity that it seems to have with allergy? In this oscillation, can we somehow see a continuity or do the observed cases only constitute a series in terms of probabilities? What is at stake in this uncertainty is nothing less than the end of a categorical confinement in partial "psychic" or "somatic" processes and systems.

Chapter 6
A New Starting Point

Abstract For a new conception of the concept of somatic, our theoretical model incorporates the contributions of relational psychosomatics, a theory that is explained and justified. First, unlike the Freudian model, our model integrates the intersubjective dimension of hypochondria that is the intersubjective dimension of psychosomatics. Then, we explain how the concept of projection can be extended, consistent with the theory of relational psychosomatics. The Body is also referred to as the potential to project. We explain how these concepts are integrated into a multidimensional model. We detail it and use it to explain the dynamics of symptom formation with a system of equivalences and transformations: depending on the nature of the dimension in which the impasse resulting from the failure of repression affects the subject, different psychical or somatic symptoms appear. We present the emerging new conception of hypochondria.

Moving beyond with new tools that are not the result of a preference but which, included in a theoretical model, nevertheless emerge from clinical experience where they actually find their true definition, this is the fundamental question that is necessarily asked by the project to really think hypochondria, which then turns into the project of a general theory of the body. The previous achievements of our reflection indeed reveal a plural way beyond the Freudian somatization model, multiple overflows seeming to echo each other to end up in a single question: what conceptualization can we identify to understand what happens in the body, symptom endowed with a symbolic value or not, that paradoxically does not take place in the body, but always in the relation to the other person?

This formulation immediately questions an elaboration process to be specified which might be defined as the search for a set of alternative hypotheses (Feyerabend 1975, p.22) to enable a reading of what contradicts the "obliged thinking." Work of negation above all, whose first expression is its search for a missing conceptualization, a conceptualization that can be formulated from the blind spots in literature, and that Feyerabend named "counterinduction," that is attempt to break the familiar circle (Feyerabend 1975, p.22).

M. Derzelle, *Towards a Psychosomatic Conception of Hypochondria*,
DOI: 10.1007/978-3-319-03053-1_6,
© Springer International Publishing Switzerland 2014

> We must invent a new conceptual system that suspends, or clashes with the most carefully established observational results, confounds the most plausible theoretical principles, and which introduces perceptions that cannot form part of the existing perceptual world (Feyerabend 1975, p.22).

The understanding of hypochondria therefore implies going beyond the Freudian model in the following major directions:

- Moving beyond it from the clinical point of view, where the cases observed are always mixed. Synchrony always replaces Diachrony (part I, 3b, II).
- Moving beyond it from the epistemological point of view, which both dismisses "Psychic" and "Somatic" as "pure" categories that are as such only absolutely mythical. Hypochondria here meets Hysteria (part I, II, 1).
- Moving beyond it from the metapsychological point of view, where the unconscious as a relationship to another person is substituted to a conception of energetic nature. Functioning is included in a situation (part III, introduction).

6.1 Symptom Pathology, Relational Pathology

Finding a starting point that enables to think hypochondria, as required by clinical observation, as a relational pathology, is probably the first requirement. For the situation identified as a triple objective, subjective, and theoretical impasse may only remain a prevented thought as long as we keep stubbornly reasoning with the Freudian model of the psychic apparatus designed as a perfect geometric object, tightly closed and existing in itself even before entering a relationship.

> How can we analyze the terms in which we habitually express our most simple and straightforward observations, and reveal their presuppositions? The answer is clear: we cannot discover it from the inside. We need an external standard of criticism (Feyerabend 1975, p.22).

The abandonment of the purely psychological vertex, which is that of an intrapsychic pathology, may however be carried out only on condition of a double statement: first that the doctor really cannot do anything—impasse on the therapeutic level duly noted—and then that this impotence is not a dismissal finding its arguments in a failing science or the vagaries of a subjectivity impossible to inscribe in the medical system—impasse in terms of thought duly noted. On these two conditions, the issues of the impasse can be formulated sanctioning a break with the strictly medical perspective that presides over all the readings in terms of description, symptoms or operation. Indeed, all assume a completed object, an enclosed space that is the place for internal processes, whose signs ordered in the discourse of the master (Clavreul 1978, p.163), have the dreaded particularity to exclude the subjectivity of their author as well as that of the one who listens. This expresses the extreme collusion between the analytic discourse for which

> hypochondria must be right, organic changes must be present in it (Freud 1914, p.83),

and where the symptom therefore refers to something formulable as a syndrome or disease, and the traditional medical discourse that dooms the patient to silence to and only hears symptoms. Moreover, in *On Narcissism: an Introduction*, the contiguity with the Bodily vividly appears in the order of the text. The reformulation of the situation as an observed impasse breaks this proximity: as objective examination does not stop complaint, the therapist's impossibility of action is the first step of a thought of the relationship.

The usual and repeated use, in literature, of the medical model, whether its approach is semiotics, diagnosis or clinical pictures, prognosis or therapeutic, can only divert from this intersubjective dimension specific to hypochondria as a radical belief. This is important because as it exclusively sees a pathology of symptoms, this model shares, implicitly, the same assumption as the Freudian model: a possible patient-physician encounter as nonrelation between two closed systems. This postulation that culminates in Freud when hypochondria is seen as an involution, i.e., reactivation of a primary narcissism considered from the angle of a genetic stage, underlies medical clinical practice from side to side. This basic assumption, taken over by Jean Clavreul in *The Medical Order* (Clavreul 1978) down to its smallest details indeed influences the possibility of a naming of these symptoms: the doctor speaks as a representative of objectivity which he guarantees; and the patient can only be an interlocutor as long as he submits to the medical order, i.e., only accepts a normality that says a health to recover (Clavreul 1978, pp.126–127). In both cases the exclusion of their respective subjectivities is considered possible, and any series of symptoms that seem indecisive are rejected into this inferior class. But there is more: as we pointed it, actual neuroses can only be maintained and defined by Freud in his thought by a surprising negativity in an approach which is not that of analysis. For, finding the support of a semiotics fading under the action of reality, they ask a serious and important question: that of an import into psychoanalysis of a founding model that is foreign to it. The latter is, of course, the medical model, as shown in the reference to the theoretical movement wherein their objectification lies. Justification of the sexual etiology of neuroses, articulation between medicine and psychoanalysis, they support the metapsychological elaboration of the Psychoneurotic. Clearly contemporary of the idea of propping sexual drives on ego drives, they are in fact invoked again during the later "discovery" of narcissism: as if their theoretical preservation allowed a definition of auto-eroticism referred to an amount of excitement in a purely somatic actuality, as well as a definition of narcissism. Propping of the psychoanalytic approach on an etiologic, pathogenic, therapeutic medical approach: sort of melting pot of a prevalidation where the major dimension of the relationship is missing.

Thinking hypochondria as relational requires therefore to conceive a model that is not thought in terms of psychic apparatus, because if we posit, using the medical method, fully individual separated subjects, having the status of an object for each other, this would mean considering that the model that we need is already built and that the problem of its constitution is already settled. Besides, this model coexists in Freud with clinical facts that contradict it. Two in particular should be emphasized: on the one hand, the existence of telepathy, existence also suspected by Ferenczi (Ferenczi 1932, pp.105–139), who seems to attest that the unconscious, immediately, communicates with the other person to whom it is open; on the other hand, the fact that the individual is always necessarily associated with the social "in this extended but entirely justifiable sense, (Freud 1921, p.69)" social which precedes him and even prepares him since the individual is first expected, so that individual psychology seems an abstraction compared to relation. Who cares! Solipsism remains side by side with its denial in the Freudian doctrine!

> To find the possibility of a relationship between humans, they invent solutions that will exacerbate the difficulty rather than resolve it; they will involve, for example identification, that is the crushing of dissimilarities. If one says, to meet a possible objection, that differentiation will be the result of the multiplication of identifications, we should admit that this is a curious detour, because what would difference emerge from and what variety would be likely in the multiplication of the Identical? In the same perspective, freedom can never have another face than of absolute independence because all influences deteriorate it. Poor Narcissus who, evading drowning, will risk paranoia!

> Would not it be wiser, since he is an animal, i.e., a psychic somatic being, to assume that the human being too makes light of opposites, that he is from the principle an individual in connection with his dissimilar fellows as well as with the world that surrounds him, that what he is subjected to is the basis of his being and his freedom, finally that in him, as living, everything can circulate and be exchanged? Both theoretical and practical consequences will appear if one wonders how a psyche that is soma works (Roustang 1970, p.12).

François Roustang formulates the same problematics, answering it by the primacy of relation. Echo of the hypothesis of Sami-Ali giving a foundation to our thinking, derived of psychosomatic clinical observation: the other starting point is relation.

> The original relationship, founder of the entire psychosomatic functioning, and that I conceive as a relationship previous to, from intrauterine life, the very terms that it connects (Sami-Ali M 1990, p.77).

Neither subject nor object, but what produces them.

6.2   Thinking the Somatic Differently

This proposal is the basic methodological requirement if we are to think hypochondria as a relation whose singular trait is to be paradoxical, interspace which looks like insolubility and whose only constant point seems to be that the complainant, whatever he does, feels necessarily doomed; but it is laden with metapsychological consequences. On the one hand, the unconscious is redefined as a relation to the other person, its conception as an energy tank being in contradiction with numerous facts; on the other hand, primary narcissism can no more be seen as a genetic category marking one of the moments of the individual evolution of what is called relation to the object, to which, multiple and diverse, the various avatars of the same regression would provide access: it becomes a problem, the one of being relationless necessarily inside a relationship. Hypochondria, as long as it operates in this mode, must therefore be referred to behaviors appeared in a specific relationship which was also a nonrelationship. Relation with a mother present by her absence.

Then a problem remains: the metapsychological problem of the constitution of the object, outside the Freudian psychic apparatus model, i.e., the definition of the conditions of its existence at the same time as a subject. On this point, the Freudian intuition articulating dream with projection, making the latter the possibility of object creation by the subject through splitting, combined with the hypothesis of Sami-Ali for whom the Imaginary, which is projection, is literally a vital function aimed at founding health and disease consistent with the early mother–child relationship, which has mediated its very constitution (Sami-Ali 1990, p.2), help us to formulate our personal thought. As this theoretical perspective, alternative procedure more in line with facts, is the one we have globally adopted it is no doubt useful to first sketch it (Derzelle and Gorot 1991). There are two essential theoretical landmarks. The first one, conceptual, is the foundation of this conception: projection is the synonymous of the Imaginary, has a biological value, and is the major and principal axis for the understanding of somatizations. The second one, of general heuristic value, allows a new conception of the Somatic, in the form of a multidimensional model including psychopathology, or repression failure pathology, and the pathology linked to the function of the Imaginary, that can be accompanied with organic symptoms when it is faced with an impasse situation: it is the formulation of a negative correlation between projection and a particular somatization affecting the Real body.

However, what is meant by projection? Psychological as much as organic concept, applicable to a wide range of phenomena ranging from normal to pathological, it refers to a process of unconscious and essentially imaginary nature involving the subject and the outside world, following the setting in motion of a retrograde movement that gives him typical traits. Projection then first means the Imaginary as opposed to the Real and which, if it includes Dream, even before the Real emerges, includes all its equivalents as well which let conscious, preconscious, and unconscious operation prevail to very different degrees in other contexts than sleep: fantasy, delusion, daydream, game, illusion, belief, uncanny, transference, affect, and hallucination, etc. Through a comprehensive modification of the relationship where the meaning of the perceived is modified, the world now plays the role of *analogon* of the ego, or simply of a part of the ego. Similarly to a spatial presence, all the external reality becomes an occult background where multiple figures of the Imaginary stand out. Far from being a defense mechanism as proposed by the analytic theory that confuses it with displacement, identification, and also transference, projection is therefore a primitive function of the developing psychic apparatus, where, below it, the reviviscence of a common psychotic background, which does not necessarily coincide with the presence of a psychotic structure, emerges. Expression of the radical noncoincidence of the subject with himself, the projective process thus expresses the fundamental fact of taking oneself for another person. Even though this mistake is attenuated and modified perhaps by the introduction of the emergence of the Real, it exists as a nostalgia of origins. The body is then above all revealed as an original capability of projection apt to endless repetitions, elusive in itself but that can be identified and in a way guessed through its effects, that is, through body images on the perceptive or imaginary level. So, far below the subject–object polarity classically evoked, a very ambiguous background still persists beyond differentiation: communication comes close to communion. Within the early mother–child relationship, place of incorporation of all automatisms, we then understand that delusion will be in proportion to the relational vacuum.

Second basic concept of this overall coherent perspective: the existence of a negative correlation between projection and a somatization of the real body. This formulation that should be demonstrated again whenever the concrete question of organic disease arises within clinical observation, and that, more than the escape toward dualism, allows the conception of everything that evades through very partial manifestations, must be connected to the renewal by Sami-Ali of the issue of the link between psychosis and allergy in *Le Visuel et le Tactile* in a unified theoretical perspective (Sami-Ali 1984). If the experience of the body is conceived in an essential dialectical opposition between the Real body and the Imaginary body—through which psychosomatics is delimited—it is therefore permissible to think that the psychotic projective predominance disrupts the whole psychosomatic operation, dramatically strengthening the immune system of the body. An enigmatic common finding is meaningful: the psychotic seldom suffer from organic diseases. What can we learn from the articulation of the usually partitioned fields of knowledge that are psychosis and allergy? The personalities prone to allergy are very characteristically in a relationship of extreme proximity to other people, proximity evoking a distress of not being able, as a face, to recognized oneself as different from the other person and, correlatively, to necessarily have the face of the other. This distress encompasses allergy itself, dependence on the other with respect to immunity, whose return is due to the fact that illusion fails to produce a unique face. But if projection is set in motion and if dependence gets absorbed in a manic agitation or delusion, allergy typically ceases immediately. Psychosis succeeds where allergy fails, taking away organicity: the allergic crisis appears only when projective action weakens. Multiple, cyclic, irregular operation which remains a potentiality and affects the immunity of the body. Projection has thus a biological value that explains this heuristically valuable negative correlation: when in an impasse situation, the unthinkable conflict becomes insoluble, projection being unable of any development, somatization then replaces regression, has a literal meaning and affects the Real body. We must then wonder if this model allows to conceptualize the oscillation pointed above between hypochondria and allergic symptoms.

6.3 Hypothesis

First observation: our model enables to think any pathology as a combination that equally includes the mode of operation of the concerned subjects as well as the situations, elaborable or not but always conflicting which they had to face. If the current nosography distinguishes four types of psychic operation, i.e., neurotic, psychotic, perverse, and operational, that disassociate Psyche from Soma and refuse to see man in his unity, the theoretical model used here indeed seeks, for each case, to locate and identify the fundamental operating mode, either imaginary or not, as a way to evaluate the projective equipment which a subject may use to confront a problematic external situation. Two axes of operation emerge, giving rise to three forms of Pathology, according to repression and its destiny. Failure of repression inseparable of the obliged symptomatic formation, successful repression inseparable of the "banal" personality formation (Sami-Ali 1980, p.77–138), alternation of failed and successful repression: these three distinct operation modes are defined by their relationship to the Imaginary but only prove to be really pathological when faced with a situation of impasse. First of the two great modes of human psychic operation, failed repression is probably one which is best-known because it corresponds to the psychopathology of the Freudian field. The failure of repression in this case establishing continuity with the Imaginary, somatization concerns the Dream body, reversible symptoms having a primary meaning. It occurs in two different forms depending on whether the conflict to solve includes or excludes contradiction itself. If it includes it, the impasse specific to psychosis, once constituted, absorbs the Real body. If it excludes it on the contrary, hysteria appears, positively correlated with somatization of the Imaginary body. The allergic structure must be added, that is also essentially governed by a projection tirelessly working to reduce the terms of the contradiction. The being of the allergic being to be identical, the projective work is a creation reducing the faces to an identical face, that is indifferently oneself as much as the other person. When difference rushes in at times of crisis, the allergic reaction then depends on a projection failing to turn the other person into a single image which is self-image.

In addition to this operation mode underpinned by projection, essentially or accidentally, there is however another operation mode, where character traits replace symptoms and pathology becomes organic: question raised by Freud but remained unanswered in the context of strict psychopathology, it is the continuous and successful repression of the function of the subjective Imaginary in favor of an extreme social adaptation in which, without being able to deny itself in its object, subjectivity is denied by its object. Triumph of the Banal, of the Mundane, of the Neutral, of the Literal. Whether it is a very temporary repression, for a simple break that must come to an end, or an extremely durable repression that could coincide with a whole life, the process remains completely the same: as if following an implicit injunction which prohibits its use, projection was suddenly put out of the game. If this injunction continues, is internalized, maintains repression long enough to induce a permanent modification of the operation mode, the absence of dreams and equivalents then marks the perfect success of repression. Success that cannot take place without a total alteration of character: with concealment of oneiric life, interest in the whole Imaginary disappears, making place for a vacuum quickly filled by an overinvestment of reality. Deserted by dream, the subject is only inhabited by its oblivion while, in character formation, a totally narcissistic relationship begins, to an instance which bars subjectivity, under its least integrable form probably because the Imaginary gives the subject, as in return, the feeling of being and of being adapted in accordance with norms, agreed to by others who are an anonymous maternal figure, integrated in a universe made of rules. Subject and Object no more exist here because they are one with the body superego. Sort of equivalent of a first projection prohibiting all projections, the latter is the internalized instance responsible for the constant double task of repressing the function of the Imaginary and substituting to it, adherence to standards, the ambient conformism of social functioning. Moral instance certainly, that says what must be but which is, at the same time highly corporeal as if any action could actually be done on the body and even through the body being turned into a functional body whose Imaginary is concealed, obliterated.

Successful repression, failed repression. The argument developed by Sami-Ali, besides it opens to another pathology, has the essential advantage of not being only reduced to the functioning: it fits in a situation whose logical structure must be taken into account, in order to understand somatization as the result of a combination of these two levels of factors, which can be ordered and arranged in several ways. An almost a priori deduction follows, made of associations which in turn are based on the Imaginary and the absence of imagination, on-contradiction, and noncontradiction. There can be multiple shades, however two great major forms of pathology basically emerge from them, they are determined, with consideration to the Imaginary, by the failure or success of an identical repression that conditions the terms in which the conflict, the external event, is expressed. Somatization and elaboration are the two major futures of the encounter of a projective equipment or its absence, at a given time, in a given situation. If maintaining the relationship with the Imaginary offers, during a conflict, the possibility of some sort of compromise between a ban and an instinctual desire by what neurotic symptom, the repressed, comes to return, which has a symbolic value, the negative relations to the Imaginary operated through repression when it is successful indeed seem to exclude any possible mediation, turning any situation into an impasse: the easy alternative of the neurotic conflict turns into an absolute alternative, pure contradiction resembling a cul-de-sac in which the person locks himself and which is hopeless. The total exclusion of the Imaginary then seems to create the conditions for a pathology affecting the Real body, diverging on this point from psychosis with which however it undoubtedly shares the same starting point, namely the contradiction of a situation of impasse. With this difference that psychosis is a final attempt to think the unthinkable, to think it notwithstanding and despite thought. The psychotic outcome is therefore a transposition of the terms of the conflict, a sort of incorporation. In this, it brings back to the Imaginary body: it shields from somatization.

What is demonstrated through such a vision—theoretical model which is both in continuity with Freudianism, to first reflect the mechanism at work in the psychoneuroses that are considered as having a meaning, and also detached from it as it refuses to see in a pathology affecting the Real body either a possible variant of actual neurosis marked with a quasi consubstantial negativity, or a form of hysterical conversion actually assimilating organic syndrome to the resurfacing of a symbolic repressed content-, is that the Imaginary determines, negatively and positively, the whole of psychosomatic dynamics. Health and disease find their basis there to the extent that they fall within an overall process, psychosomatic, governed by symptomatic transformation. This variability, which allows to follow the plural deployment of a pathology outside the "psychic" and "somatic" partitioning, introduces at the same time the continuity of a mode of operation often partially understood. If projection is the main axis, it is because it already has a biological value and is the indicator, at one point, of the whole economy of a subject, overall economy that is psychosomatic.

We therefore hypothesize the following, in an attempt to actually think hypochondria thanks to a different conceptual system:

1. Belief in a mysteriously affected body including in its cipher a relationship to the other person, hypochondria, projective process, homologous more than prelude to paranoia, is the elaboration of an impasse situation that reveals that a previous operation mode that has become the prevalent adaptive attitude, is inoperative.

2. Impasse transcended as it has been incorporated into the elaboration of the unthinkable, hypochondria needs to be situated in the context of somatization, impassable impasse offered to thought in a typical symptomatic oscillation. From somatic it becomes mental, like the passage pointed in our examples from allergy to the hypochondriac crisis as if the failure-achievement of the first triggered the beginning of psychosis.

Chapter 7
Hypochondria, Projective Parenthesis

Abstract We demonstrate that the concept of projection gives a positive content to hypochondria and constitutes the missing link between the diverse forms of this disorder. We explain how relational psychosomatics defines projection as a process born from and iteratively going back to the stage of undifferentiation, before the possibility for the subject to integrate alterity. We explain why the question of alterity is crucial in hypochondria and other psychic and somatic symptoms. The Schreber case, as well as our clinical observations, exemplify symptom equivalences and transformations, as well as the conceptual relation between hypochondria and paranoia. This leads to a new hypothesis: hypochondria as the limited elaboration of an impasse.

Projection really seems to be the conceptualization that we seek. As it gives hypochondria a positive content, where we can find the answer to one of our questions—how to think a designation that the Freudian system presents as negative?—it turns it into a form of the Imaginary, a manifestation of failed repression, whose proximity with paranoia, its homologue, must be noticed, limited in time and to the body however, its proximity to hysteria too from which it differs by form only but not by function. But projection adds some even more valuable aspects to the question of the body:

- Psychological as much as biological concept, it allows to think beyond the Freudian model of somatization, considering both health and disease as moments in a larger development. It is thus possible to include in the analysis of paranoia, known as "pure psychosis," hypochondriac and organic phenomena as phases of a long psychosomatic process. It is thus possible to include in the analysis of "princeps" hysteria, organic as well as psychotic phenomena (Sami-Ali 1987, pp.32–61) as signs of a symptomatic variability. "Psychic" sometimes follows "Somatic," but "Psychic" sometimes follows "Psychic," and "Somatic" sometimes follows "Psychic." In such a sequence, a negative equivalence relation emerges between psychic and somatic symptoms as if they occupied, within the same set, two perfectly symmetrical opposite positions. All are parentheses in an operation mode. And hypochondria is thus an episode.

M. Derzelle, *Towards a Psychosomatic Conception of Hypochondria*,
DOI: 10.1007/978-3-319-03053-1_7,
© Springer International Publishing Switzerland 2014

- Synonymous with the Imaginary as apt to a double correlation, it allows deduction as an a priori of the finite set of Pathology, deduction supported by clinical experience. The absence of a general theory of the body, of which the absence of a status of hypochondria seems a variant, is then solved in a relevant way, the relation to the Imaginary determining the strictly hysterical somatization as well as the nonhysterical organic one. One and the other constituting the extremes of a continuum-spectrum where, depending on either the Imaginary or its repression prevails at a given time, the various somatization phenomena are aspects of the same substantive process: exit the epistemological break. Passages from the Real body to the Imaginary body that say that there cannot be one Static but two dialectical functions instead, depending on whether projection applies to the body or not. Hypochondria as a projective parenthesis?

7.1 Projection, the Missing Conceptualization

As it is a repetition of automatisms acquired in a relationship, i.e., this early mother–child relationship whose typical character is to preexist the terms that it connects, projection taken as a thinking tool basically prevents hypochondria from being reduced to the single objective description of a nosophobia or to the interpretation of painful but mysterious sensations: therefore its study depends on the search for the meanings of a typical relationship, without which one cannot speak of hypochondria. But can we conceive this repetition? What sort of impasse at the level of relationship does hypochondria, as projective attempt, try to overcome, sort of relationship established on the model of childhood and with a background that is free from differentiation? Sami-Ali answers the first metapsychological question, in *On projection,* incorporating Freud's successive observations:

> It is as if the projective process tirelessly got back to this crucial phrase during which the distinction between the ego and the outside world occurs... When this move backwards is made, it is not limited to the reproduction of a previous situation, more or less transcended, because each dive into undifferentiation causes significant economic changes. Through this contact restored with the first psychic reality a new energy distribution between the inside and the outside develops. The ego introjects what does not yet belong to it or what it is separated from, as well as it projects its specific contents or the contents that it has already appropriated by introjection. It thus creates a continual back and forth motion that communicates its creator rhythm to psychic life. And however, everything suggests that projection is possible only because it was possible once for the first time. It seems to endlessly repeat an initial possibility, once given never to be withdrawn. There is a temporal attachment point indicating the limit of the regressive movement in projection. Attachment point which has the remarkable property to be part of no particular clinical picture but instead to appear to be the essential condition that allows the ego to exist in the world (Sami-Ali 1970, pp.189–190).

The "same thing" that is repeated is not a datum that can be apprehended in immediacy: it includes perceptual content and also gets back to the relational form that presides over and conveys the process. The cause of the impasse still has to be explained.

Way of thinking where the unconscious prevails constantly turning the subject into objects, of which nocturnal dream is a modality and which questions the polarity postulated between the inside and the outside, projection also sheds a light on hypochondria because it is not only the transformation of a perception of something internal into something external recognized as such: it is also the belief that it is an absolute objective reality. Totally unable to take his distance from himself as soon as he projects, the subject trusts all the perceptions that impose on him in an illusory way. Because projection is an act of faith whereby the leap into the Imaginary happens (Sami-Ali 1970, p.147). An Imaginary that supplants the Real where a complete faith, in terms of desire, can turn the world into a de-real background where internal perceptions are projected. The hypochondriac, however, is singular because projection remains limited to his body experienced as sick and to the other person, the all-powerful/powerless caregiver whose meeting is at the heart of the suffering being. What matters from the start is being, not knowing. All that is perceived is at the same time felt. Even time undergoes a characteristic major distortion. Internalization is the first act: the subject lives to the rhythm of medicines, exemptions, internal progressions, clocks that regulate him out of "objective" time. Because if the latter cannot be abolished, it becomes lacunar, resisting the anamnesis of any previous somatic reality. The fading of the past is revealed by the "present" of the consultation. The future also is denied, at least in its dimension of project. "I will die of cancer"; "I will lose my mind": the future is interrogative, act of supreme faith in body affection. As the time of dream, present is the only possibility, an absolute present that seems limitless and merges with the presence of a body which gives time all its points of reference. An ambiguous chronicity results, guarantee against mortality and also great impossibility to live in the sense that living is living in time. Painful endurance whose disjointed, discontinuous and in a way materialized time ignores the present said to be authentic, hypochondria is a dyschronic chronicity. Eternal present: time of accomplishment, of dreams, of belief.

Paradoxically defined by Henri Ey as essential form of human existence (Ey 1950, p.480), hypochondria finds its truth there in the sense that it releases the projective kernel immanent to the whole human nature, kernel that is synonymous with the Imaginary, with the Unconscious as originary, in fact. Common psychotic background, comparable to dream, also likely of an always renewed distribution of self and objects, projection here is form of existence revealing its anchorage in corporeality. So says Henri Ey:

> By its very structure, hypochondria is an illusion, and the problem of hypochondria is only one aspect of hallucinatory and delusional projection. But the specificity of illusion is precisely that it is experienced at the same time on the registers of the Imaginary and the Real. The reality contained by hypochondria is nothing but the very reality of our body belonging to our 'world', it is not that of the corporeality of a certain part or function of the body (which enters our consciousness as an object only in exceptional or unhealthy conditions), but this experience 'by what I am my body' and that binds 'my' body to 'me' in the relationship of 'having'. It is the perfect disposition of my body that goes beyond my control in hypochondria and what I feel in my body then is an event and an accident happening there in spite of me and against me (Ey 1950, p.479).

No surprise that hypochondria is, in literature, highly extravagant, unclassified, a neurosis or even a psychosis, characterized by a kind of ubiquity. Structure of existence become form of existence, it says that the body is a power of projection, from which health and disease may be inferred, whether conflict finds a way toward elaboration or not. Multipurpose transverse designation, it speaks of the Real as well as the Imaginary body. Hypochondria, the problem, in the Freudian corpus, with its tenacious appearance of continuum, has therefore a power of truth: it shows that another model can be rethought, taking projection for its major axis. Many of the contradictions of a double existence of subject and object, of included and including, that constantly attracts us on the side of anxiety and disease, find their solution in it. Hypochondria, the problem: food for thought...

7.2 The Schreber Case and its Hypochondriac Episode

The fundamental contribution of the use of the concept of projection is, undoubtedly, that it allows to think hypochondria first as an episode taken in the deployment of a pathology governed by symptomatic transformation. In the Schreber case (Freud 1911), it appears to be the first phase of a long process which, although interspersed with periods of relief, evolves into a paranoid psychosis, finally, peaking shortly before the subject's death, into a chronicity and a cardiovascular type pathology that finally proves fatal. Already interpretable as a delusion of the body, neither simple in its structure, nor actual by its cause, the hypochondriac episode is supported by a projection from one end to the other, preventing that can change, against evidence and against the doctor, the belief in a mysteriously affected body. What to say then but that the Freudian principle which considers hypochondria as the actual core of paranoia seems inapplicable? What to say then but that it is, from the beginning, the homologue of paranoia, of inherently projective essence, with this difference that as it is limited spatially and temporally Schreber was able to recover "cured"? Everything obviously depends on what we mean by "cured," which seems here to correspond to the designation, at a specific time of the evanescence of symptomatology, itself inextricably linked to a true change in global or psychosomatic functioning which makes health and illness appear as abstractions designating, for lack of a better term, the succession of various symptomatic sets defined by their relationship to the Imaginary. No doubt for example that the hypochondriac ideas of Schreber really disappeared, return of the repressed leaving a scene which, however, never remained deserted for long. Everything happens as if hypochondria had suddenly made breach in a functioning that is specific to successful repression, which then resumes, absorbing the hypochondriac symptoms by the establishment of a new and as reinforced personality organization. Re-organization more than organization of what existed before the failed repression and which can define "normal" personality, referred to as the absence of symptoms. When this functioning resumes, because of another new repression, hypochondria looks like an incident that it seems to put in parentheses.

A circular causality is therefore observed, made of broken lines, where repression follows repression, interrupted only by projective phases of which hypochondria is an incident (see Fig. 7.1). Its healing is just a successful repression, an end put by character functioning to a seemingly accidental projective flash: its result is a paranoid character much more rigid than the previous one, marked by distrust, but free however from organic symptoms. Its role is essential

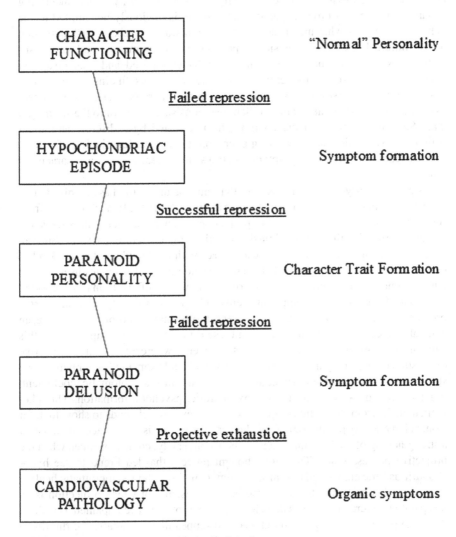

Fig. 7.1 Underlying dynamic situation in the Schreber case

for body anxiety: it completely stops it as it replaces it, but falls apart, a few years later, in the paranoid delusions. Remarkable fact however: if this incident has disturbed the previous functioning, the latter both seems to be cause and effect of constant repression. Cause, first of all, because once it has been adopted as a background attitude against all drives, the characterial repression continues according to the same pattern in which the failure of repression is followed by a repression supposed to be a remedy. But this functioning is also the effect of repression itself, because as it operates in contact with drives, it incorporates them too, at least partially, to better repel them in a second movement. So that a sustainable compromise can take place between repressed content and repression, in which the repressing instance prevails, working tirelessly. This underlying dynamic situation, of obvious paradigmatic value, is obviously not limited to the Schreber case: it is what underlies, in an essential way, any character functioning whose failure leaves room, outside hypochondria, for numerous and varied somatizations which in turn regress, are more widely spaced and then disappear when characterial repression prevails (see Fig. 7.2). This finding leads to two observations. The first one lies in the assertion that there is undoubtedly no pre-psychotic condition as the healing of Schreber consists in a return to the *status quo ante*. Second assertion: on the contrary, he is affected by a discrete and silent pathology, psychotic character taking over from the normal functioning of before. The absence of organic symptoms betrays the presence of a characterial repression.

As paranoia, psychosomatic disorder that must be understood as an episode in a development in which projection that works as dream holds the Real body away from somatizations, hypochondria, as of projective essence, perfectly illustrates the negative correlation that we mentioned, projection having a biological value. Such an observation in appearance harmoniously agrees with the Freudian idea of a kind of perfect narcissistic equivalence between hypochondria and somatic disease, in a purely economic perspective. Our point of view however differs. If, in three reported cases out of four, somatic complaint seems to begin immediately after an allergic problem, if according to doctors negative reports often have a morbid organic fate, an equivalence can be established between these different sets of symptoms, but this equivalence is given as negative: psychosis succeeds where allergy fails, projective exhaustion opens on organic expression. "Psychic" and "somatic" occur here as two strictly symmetrical positions: equipped with a same symptomatic coefficient, organic affection appears in lieu of any neurotic, psychotic formation. This phenomenon, far from "somatic complacency," however which tends to show that, far from being a purely psychological mechanism, projection is always accompanied by a strengthening of the immune system which, conversely, come to weaken when the projective process fades. The same thought process that led Freud to see hypochondria as little elaborated thus also led him to misjudge how symptomatic healing worked: in his system, a theory of the body is missing, of which projection is an inseparable feature. Schreber's delusions, as they grow, are accompanied as well by the same process, causing the spontaneous disappearance of an allergic rhinitis in conjunction with a resistance so exceptional that Schreber can feel "immortal." This

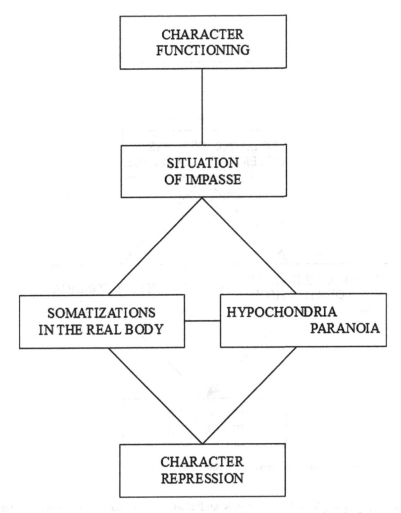

Fig. 7.2 Underlying dynamic situation in the case of failure of character functioning

shows that what we have here is not the elaboration of hypochondria, as argued by Freud, but a situation of impassable impasse, where somatization in the Real body constitutes the other term of the alternative.

7.3 The Limited Development of an Impasse

Once its projective nature, and then its positive link to the Imaginary, have been identified, hypochondria in a way acquires a metapsychological basis as it operatively very concretely involves, in clinical practice, a typical symptomatic

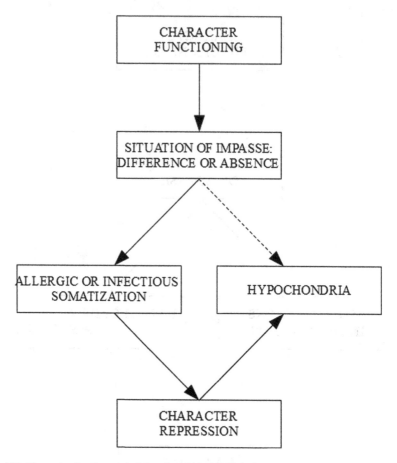

Fig. 7.3 Dynamic situation underlying the observed clinical cases

variability where "Psychic" absorbs and changes "Somatic." Observation here tends to go beyond it, revealing the profound unity of the phenomenon whose definition can be articulated around several proposals. We will only present some of them, derived from the dynamic situation underlying the four previously narrated clinical cases (see Fig. 7.3), so that they can be viewed, described, interpreted through a relevant replacement procedure. The following remarks apply:

- In our four cases, hypochondria imperturbably makes a breach in a character functioning where the prevailing process in the impasse situation is allergic somatization, which marks the emergence of the Different in a world where the implacable logic of identity only reigns. Indeed, the latter characterizes the relational work, said characterial, as well as the work of allergy phenomena (Sami-Ali 1987, p.21).

- This functioning which is not inherently pathogenic, but cuts short conflict and its implications, becomes pathogenic when the subject is suddenly totally and radically unable to neutralize absence and difference. These take by surprise a relational game where contradiction is excluded. The impasse says the unthinkable of a situation uniting the Identical with its negation.

  Allergy invariably seems to appear in such a situation, indicating the inability to reduce, to overcome contradiction. Sporadic symptoms in the form of a regression where the subject draws on its biological resources, it restores with the other person, often as in childhood, a relationship broken by the sudden eruption of an acute perception of difference.

- Another possible term of the alternative, hypochondria begins where allergy fails, having a common starting point with it.

In front of contradiction, that allergy resolves on the biological level by a restoration of the almost identical, psychosis embeds it in its own thought which is an elaboration of the unthinkable: there, the question of the other person can no longer arise.

Conceived as a relational pathology, that is as the result of a combination of operation mode and "life event" of confrontational value, on an equal basis, hypochondria connotes therefore three essential facts. It is first the revelation of an earlier adapted state collapsing because it cannot tolerate to integrate, in a system insistently characterized by the total repression of the Imaginary, a situation of distress or conflict generating a situation of impasse. It is then the symptomatic equivalent of a somatization of allergic type, with this major difference that the first begins where the second ends, total conversion work that turns a contradiction into Identical, causing an allergic bout which expresses the failure of a unique relationship as a result of the emergence of the Different. As paranoia, but limited to the body, it is therefore the development of an unthinkable situation by the integration of contradiction in a thought whose structure is changed, putting in question the essential principles that govern the latter in its formal logic. Far from being limited to purely physical symptoms, as the theory of actual neuroses explains it (Freud 1973, p.365), hypochondria is therefore basically a pathology of thought: born from the relationship to the other person as different, contradiction disappears at the same time as the other person. A continuity thus seems to be established between character, allergy, hypochondria, around one same extreme proximity to the other person, unsustainable intrusive presence of the mother which, historically, is first and foremost a face. But there are some differences, which prevent them from be totally similar. If, in character as in allergy, conflict is excluded in a same approach reducing all beings to a unique one, the relationship involving two people, whose absence is typical of character where the subject is only relationship from self to self image, is present in allergy where the real problem is the existence of self relatively to the other person. If, in allergy as in hypochondria, the other is projectively an imaginary being, the former succeeds where the latter fails, these two eventualities are like the two stages of the same fundamental problem. If, in character as in hypochondria, the other person can only be a body superego, the projection supporting a character, that initially forbids to project, responds to the projection that invades hypochondria.

For our four cases of negative reports, a hypothesis seems therefore to emerge: belief in a mysteriously affected body including in his cipher a relationship to the other person, hypochondria, real projective process homologous to paranoia, is the elaboration of a situation of impasse where self-identity is at stake, creating through projection, similarly to dream a reality that is restoration of a relationship to another on the model of childhood, that is a relationship in the form of a paradox. In question here is a situation where only the inner meaning is important, support of a projection that is the repetition of a reaction that has its place in a story: the relational void caused by the loss of a maternal figure experienced as all-powerful, on which the subject's identity depends through a coincidence of "be" and "must," apart from being an existential aporia because the absence of framework is harbinger of death, is also the occasion of a repetition of automatisms acquired in a relationship. An impossible approach responds to the impossible: the withdrawal of the other person, unthinkable because the feeling of existence of the subject depends on him/her, sees its emptiness filled almost instantly by a projection informing this nothingness. Everything happens as if the relational void induced by a real loss, absence or difference of a constituent object that is promise of self as body superego, suddenly automatically revived the former functioning in the same circumstances, that is in the early mother–child relationship, the need to give shape to a void which, paradoxically, confronted the child to a mother denied by a double nothingness, absent by her presence, present by her absence. As if the collapse of body superego, object of a precise initial projection laying down the prohibition of further projection (Sami-Ali 1987, p.21), resulted in the partial lifting of the latter to recreate the object as imaginary. As if a limited and single projection of an Other, all-powerful and narcissistic double, fixing the situation of impasse, gave way to another superego figure, with this major difference however that it is as the hither of body superego, that it is the paradoxical relational context in which the latter constituted in early life. As to the mother of yesterday, the subject is bound to the doctor of today in singular ways: the requirement of a cure arises concurrently with a belief of incurability, health and illness seem equivalent within a relationship of absolute dependence that has no end because it gives existence while removing it at the same time.

Chapter 8
A Different Relation to Oneself and to the Other Person

Abstract We show that difficulty to integrate alterity constitutes a fundamental element in the hypochondriac's psychosomatic dynamics. Consequently, we explain why in hypochondria, projection results in a paradoxical relationship in which the subject uses the doctor as his own double. We make use of the concepts of narcissism and distance to improve our understanding of this "uncanny" situation.

The enigma of hypochondria we focused on (See Introduction), all the more striking in the descriptions that the dimension of explanation is absent (See Sect. 1.1), can be deciphered if it is thought of differently as the actualization, in conditions other than sleep and nocturnal dreams, of what is just a variant of dream, a similar transformation of the subject into object(s) where contradiction disappears as well as the other person. Projection here supplants perception, putting an end to the splitting between Real and Imaginary, whereby the link to another is transformed, banning the very issue of alterity. The emergence of the other person as different from oneself, which is also marked by the allergic attack, therefore appearing as the equivalent of a residue of the Real impossible to transform into a dream, leads on the contrary to an oneiric material in an insomniac way in the hypochondriac: by an absolute narcissistic shift on himself, opposites objectivize, substituting the continuous movement of a spiral thought that spins around in the form of soliloquy to an alternative that rigidly imposes an unequivocal choice. By a total conversion into Identical, contradiction weaves a new logic: there is now only a single object in which the subject dissolves, coinciding there with the Imaginary that has become the Real, internal as much as external. That is to say how the lack of a theoretical status to clearly think hypochondria is linked to the underlying lack of a theoretical status identifying projection, since what is in question there is the imaginary space which is specified by magical thinking, a dynamic controlled by a fascination where the distance between subject and object fades away. This also shows how the theory of Sami-Ali that filled in this theoretical gap by giving projection a specific status that fits into a metapsychology (Sami-Ali 1970, pp.163–218), provides our study with a thinking tool thanks to which "clues" can be spotted, indicating the effect of

M. Derzelle, *Towards a Psychosomatic Conception of Hypochondria*,
DOI: 10.1007/978-3-319-03053-1_8,
© Springer International Publishing Switzerland 2014

projection where truth gives way to influence. Analogous to the concept of "uncanny" that Freud elaborated in 1914 (Freud 1919, pp.217–253), the same relationship of reciprocal inclusions presides here in what is a relationship to another person whose singular trait is to be, unknowingly, a relationship to oneself. This symmetric structure which is the structure of dream where outside and inside are equivalents, only partially invades perception: limited to the body alone, it engenders a Real that results from the duplication of the subject who ignores it and, like him, reflects the image of its double.

If contradiction disappears with the other person where projection replaces perception, transforming it into the ambiguous stooge of a drama whose only theme is self-image, this allows us to re-assess the meanings, repeatedly expressed, that remain a blind spot until projective action can explain them.

> So we now face the one who has a passion for medical knowledge, who builds his own anatomy and pathogenesis, who erects his own explanatory systems. It is both familiar and strange (with the meaning of *unheimliche*) for a physician to be confronted with his caricatured double (Delahousse and Hitter-Spinelli 1980, p.44), or:

> In this drama, the roles are sometimes assigned to a single actor, who alternately puts on and takes off his mask to talk to himself: but, more often, it is played by two people, between whom there is a similarity and a connivance so misleading that they allow these enigmatic twins, although the viewer cannot notice anything, to swap their roles (Maurel 1973, p.80).

There is always a symmetric space where the other person represents a narcissistic double, exactly as in paranoia. Three major terms seem clear, providing hypochondria with a unique structure:

(1) First, the usual object relation is replaced by the splitting of oneself into two. Projection, creation of a reality beyond oneself that is oneself, seems inseparable from a relationship to the world of an original type which is narcissism (Sami-Ali 1970, pp.75–88). It is built on the model of the ties that link the subject to his own image, where he seeks himself without even noticing that it is only a mirror. Thus hypochondria is inextricably linked to a perfect duplication of oneself in the other person, another person as mysterious and strange as the trouble that lives in the subject, disturbing him.

(2) This relationship then has the form of a paradox. Endless game where a double blindness seems in question: that of the doctor who sees nothing where the patient tells him that there is something and that of the patient who tries to suggest the existence of a conflict but who cannot see anything. It is because paradox is the verbal form of the reciprocal inclusion, the two conflicting proposals involved encasing the subject in a double word that at the slightest movement, surrounds him and tightens on him until suffocation. The "double bind" illuminates a pathology where in fact health equals illness (Sect. 3.3).

(3) This relationship, finally, is the repetition of an early relational situation, background constituent of body superego where the distortion of the maternal function, that equates "you must" with "you mustn't," confusing one with the

other and assimilating them, prevents the subject from leaving the iterative field that holds him captive. Ill, he uses the other person, the doctor, in the quest for a probable future healing. Considered not ill, he maintains this need, in the quest for a possible condition that has to be named. But if he was free from the forces that immobilize him, he probably could not exist for himself.

The instance which prohibits existence allows existence: avatar of an internal configuration where the subject can only live condemned.

Duplication of oneself, paradox, superego: a dual mother–child relationship is revealed, completely obscuring the existence of the father, where a doubly effective projection is the symmetrical response for both partners and creates an imaginary complementarity between two identical universes where everyone is in turn self, the other person, a part of the other person. Identity is imposed here with psychosis.

8.1 Intersubjective Dimension of Hypochondria

From the beginning, the encounter with the doctor is not an exterior event, it implicitly concerns what happens to the body and is located immediately in the middle of pain; the *Memoirs of My Nervous Illness* (Schreber 1903) written by Schreber clearly evidenced this, corroborated by psychiatric reports (Baumeyer 1955) which show to what extent bodily complaints, ceaselessly repeated and incomprehensible, refracted by the same interpretive scheme, are linked to a way of apprehending other people in their strangeness on an exclusive mode. Hypochondria then first appears under the typical highly narcissistic species of a singular relationship to oneself and to the other person, where the distance is nonexistent and extreme at the same time. Extreme because the other person, converted into an imaginary being, as the mother before, is considered in its absolute difference. Nonexistent yet as much because at the same time the other is perceived instead of oneself. Between these two extremes projection draws a path, centered on the object that fascinates by its proximity as by its distance, in which suffering is at stake. Concerns related to the weight of the body are thus in Schreber the main part of the "first nervous disease (Schreber 1903)," presenting a conflict entirely centered on the body and especially on what it ought to be according to a dialectic confronting the subject with the requirements of body superego. But what is involved in physical suffering is psychical functioning: things are now strange and unusual, perception drifting toward fascination. Fascination with the attitude of Schreber, as he had, in his words, in the first phase, "only favorable impressions of Professor Flechsig's methods of treatment (Schreber 1903, p.45)."

He was probably impressed, as it can sometimes happen, by an image maker, who created illusions and other pretense all the more so because his art made him "clairvoyant (Maurel 1973, p.77)." Sham character, whose acts and words are fake in a world where existence is reduced to appearance. It is because reality, which is only the coating of void and is in fact unreal, is undermined from the inside: the other person is only a split image, projected image becoming unreal as it gradually gains consistence. When existence is expressed here it is also denied: a dual knot exists which cannot be slashed. Nothing can therefore put an end to the travesty set in its scenery.

The first disease in the form of hypochondria is, therefore, not outside the field of psychosis. The experience of the body is central, determining an only spatial world (Sami-Ali 1977, pp.33–36), but the relationship to the other person indeed also allows to see there, much more than a truth problem, a problem of influence and even of dependence, that is consistently the insistent presence of a projection transforming reality. Because whether it is paranoid or belongs to conversion hysteria, projection is formed around "something" that the subject can recognize in himself but that he perceives in the other person as a problem. Others are used as a mirror, and perception is a narcissistic function excluding knowledge. What is then revealed is the real purpose, at least the intersubjective dimension of hypo-chondria as "uncanny (Sami-Ali 1977, pp.22–36)," where the falsity of the other person says his identity: it is reduplication of oneself in the other, as mysterious and strange as the trouble that possesses the subject. "Small details" seen as "unimportant" betray an object circumscribed but fleeing, projection of the Enigma and of its decryption. The other is elusive but is seized as such through trifles noticed in the Real. So hypochondria is inextricably linked to a status of "detail," specific and accurate. This status is firstly equivalent to a whole, to the object entirely divided into parts of object which are also the object, sign of a relationship of reciprocal inclusions: the "lies" of the doctor say the duplicity of an entire universe whose interpretation actually creates the reality to interpret. It is secondly what is imposed through denial as if it were a failed repression that would burst through a formula to be reversed. "Details, said Schreber, that I do not consider so important (Schreber 1903, p.45)." What means, on the contrary: things so important that even denial cannot erase them. It is finally what confirms what one pretended to ignore, that the other can have control over the body and that suffering demonstrates this power. What happens to the body is indeed supported by a relationship with the medical world, where the fate of the subject is given as a sheer dependence to the object. Place of betrayal, the detail is then also the place of conversion! Of subject into object, of inside into outside, of perception nearly into hallucination.

Everything is therefore as if, in this relational disorder, the impossibility of the subject to grasp, at the level of consciousness, what could work as a narcissistic *analogon*, was in a way caught in some "perceptions" in which consciousness is absorbed without reason and which captivate it to precisely cut it from the subject. Two details are thus retained against Professor Flechsig; Schreber claims he had used "white lies" and purposely delayed his recovery.

> Yet I could only consider it a white lie when, for instance, Professor Flechsig wanted to put down my illness solely to poisoning with potassium bromide, for which Dr. R. in S, in whose care I had been before, was to be blamed. I believe I could have been more rapidly cured of some hypochondriacal ideas by which I was preoccupied at the time, particularly

concern over loss of weight, if I had been allowed to operate the scales which served to weigh patients a few times myself _ the scales used in the University Clinic were of a particular construction unfamiliar to me (Schreber 1903, p.45).

In what Flechsig does, in total control of the Real and the body as an all-powerful mother, everything is deception. Even word is sleazy, dubious, double, in a way, and things are never there simply by themselves but on a background of unclear premonitions and intentions. Because what we can see here is the return of the repressed, noticeable in certain qualities governed by a hidden and dark causality beyond the division between subject and object.

Therefore, a general leveling of perceptual experience forcing the subject to live his relationships with the world as if he himself was an object among objects and these were not different from him (Sami-Ali 1970, p.129).

In a world where influence and evil spells prevail, primacy is given to things which, losing their exteriority, become the pretext of a power being exercised. Machines used to influence closely or remotely which are disturbing because of their distance as well as of their strange familiar closeness. The scales are a good example: object-image of the body supposed to put an end to doubt in deciding the difficult question of weight, it increases it, so that the anxiety which has already taken hold of the body becomes endless. Object-trap in which one gets lost as in a maze. The subject is radically all objects where the impasse opens a space of reflections.

8.2 The Relation to a Narcissistic Double

This very characteristic transformation of the world into a double that can be called narcissistic is an overt reduction to the Identical via metamorphosis into dreamlike material. This needs to be explained. First it is not trite to note that duplication into subject and object exactly reproduces a past dependence relationship with the other person as superego instance: tortured, sentenced, slave, manipulated, the patient of today is like the child of yesterday. The fact the other person is the support of many projections making it appear as a narcissistic double therefore seems to be the result of a first projection fixing this situation once and for all. This is to say that hypochondria is linked to a narcissism that has not been overcome and that has no need of a reactivation conventionally presented as regressive (Freud 1915[1917]a, pp.223–224): it is the fixation to the transformation of the maternal object into body superego. And everything happens as if the relational void induced by a real loss suddenly revived the former functioning in the same circumstances, that is in the early mother–child relationship, the need to give shape to a void which, paradoxically, confronted the child to a mother denied by a double nothingness. Instead of a bereavement which cannot be carried out in a system unable to integrate it, the hypochondriac tries, on the model of childhood, to give body and form to what is gaping. Repeatedly, with the doctor, a total dependence relationship restoring the infant's to his mother, alienates the subject and returns him to himself, but without himself, out of himself, objectivized (Sami-Ali 1984, p.138 note 3).

Because the other person's difference means losing an identity that is the other person's. Projectively giving his own substance to the missing object recreated as imaginary thus puts an end to a link that has deleterious effects: in addition to stopping what looks like an unlimited energetic drain, by what Different was constantly reduced to Identical, hypochondria is able to cancel the possibility of otherness even as the other is self, out of self, unknowingly, dealing with the world that has become a mirror. In the same motion any situation of impasse is banned forever because distress and conflict have no meaning here. Being a pain, hypochondria is the mourning of all pains. Being a pain, hypochondria is a pain-relieving lure. It is Narcissus looking at the water and receiving, said Bachelard,

the revelation of his identity and his duality, the revelation of his double masculine and feminine powers, and especially the revelation of his reality and his ideality (Bachelard 1947, p.34).

A second comment is needed on this point. Even if it is not seized by consciousness that only apprehends objective data whose link to the subject is completely cut off, cut where repression is completed as if only the exterior seemed to replace an experience that has become unknown, perceptual identity can be identified anyway by certain qualities that give it an exceptional emotional value. Always keeping with its source a secret link preventing it from losing its singularity, the object on which projection operates bears visible "signs" making it highly "interesting." With this in mind, we can find a meaning to the typical attitudes often noticed in somatic complainants: we can see that the object isn't perhaps as "exterior" as it seems. The existence of a projective process at work thus seems identifiable through an enigmatic presence, always fascinating and disturbing by its ambiguity and its strangeness, these features revealing that the doctor constitutes a narcissistic double. The Enigmatic first, repressed content seized by the subject as a void surrounding the fullness of being, a lacuna more real than reality, whose extreme expression regularly appears as an unavoidable feeling of inauthenticity. This is because projection of innermost data to the outside world places the subject before an unconscious expression of himself, which increases the dependence of the subject on the object. The object is no more a present being but, instead, the place of existence of another strange object, beyond control and consistency. This missing object, which yet is nothing but the subject himself ignored by himself, is therefore the hidden trigger of a series of singular events, which typically shatters usual perception. Perceiving now equates guessing and premonition is electively used to pierce the other person's opacity. Enigmatic, it is shady and elusive, hidden behind immeasurable acts and gestures. Clues, presumptions, traces, indications: these snippets of information are the only possibility when one wants to discover, as being the other people's, a truth that is only one's own. The Enigmatic here joins the Impenetrable.

The double is also fascinating, analogous to the object of passion that Freud compared several times to (Freud 1921, pp.111–116) hypnosis and showed it was a variant of it (Freud 1921, p.114). In either case, the object is extremely overrated, as idealized, attractive, to the point of "consuming the ego (Freud 1921, p.112)," attracting a huge amount of libido. However, there is no identification to the object becoming internalized, as it is not entirely external to the subject, and the object is fascinating, performing functions now deserted by the subject himself, that are judgment and reality testing. In a word everything happens here as if

the object has been put in the place of the ego ideal (Freud 1921, p.113),

fascination itself revealing an object that is part of the subject. In addition, this relationship to the fascinating object, that attracts mainly when it has positive qualities, can also tie up with objects because of their negative characteristics: they are then "ugly," "repugnant," "disgusting," but the subject is similarly attached. Thus the powerful and powerless doctor occupies the subject as a parasitic object.

Each duelist exposes himself, opposes, imposes in the sado-masochistic climate of a fascinating and perilous struggle. The referee or spectator of this duel could hardly determine which is sadistic, and which is masochistic: they are equals, ambiguous, giving care for care, blow for blow, wound for wound (Maurel 1973, p.80).

Any perception of the double indeed includes the element that Freud called "uncanny," theme that he treated exhaustively (Freud 1919), showing how the object is, at the same time, outside and inside in this case, both present and absent, strange and familiar in its ambiguity. This last results, within narcissism, from a total confusion of things and ego, return of the repressed where the usual maintained distance between "here" and "there" is lost. We then understand why Henri Maurel affirms that the interlocutor is essential:

Against all logic, we do not start with the hero; and we even delay his entry as much as possible, as the best approach to the hypochondriac, that perhaps classical psychiatry was wrong to neglect, is to consider the interlocutors… At the end of these approximations, perhaps we will eventually discover that, in the chiaroscuro of the projected shadows, we have already drawn the portrait of the subject through the mirror (Maurel 1973, p.42).

But sometimes the action is apparently lonely, the subject, disappointed by a fake doctor, irresponsible oracle of his own speech, goes, as the Misanthrope, to "a remote place" and utters in the "desert" a monologue intended for other people. The action will then involve an interlocutor and will, in a hallucinatory "detachment," autistically give voice to the organ, whose function is to keep going. This function, Word of the body, will be par excellence the excretory function, whose alternation of retention and release will set the pace of speech and organize it into an imaginary dialogue that Freud, in particular, described in President Schreber (Maurel 1973, p.80).

Chapter 9
Towards a Psychosomatic Conception of Hypochondria

Abstract We sum up and explain the theoretical and clinical contributions of this study of hypochondria. A new clinical case exemplifies them. Thanks to the psychosomatic conception of hypochondria we go in-depth into the complexity of this case to open new perspectives on hypochondria and other disorders.

Thinking hypochondria in this perspective, alternative hypothesis of a prospective nature, therefore produces new effects. Because when we question the status of the body on the basis of a multidimensional model, our research results in a new plural set of landmarks on a possible therapeutic level as well as on the technical and theoretical one which could constitute "the formula sought." These contributions are the following:

(1) In the global reflection on systems, two important findings obviously emerge:

- The study of hypochondria shattered the Freudian model based on an evolutionary organization. Transverse notion of projective nature, if hypochondria is first and foremost a belief including in its cipher a relationship to another person, it does not only defeat a notion of Actuality designed as symptoms that are purely physical, it also nullifies all two-dimensional models introducing a radical break between two dimensions of the somatic, thought in relation to transference, positively as well as negatively.
- The study of hypochondria shattered the Freudian model which was based on a purely psychological concept, pure denial from which the analytical game emanates, which is a double exclusion of reality in its social as well as biological form and to which any discourse on Actuality is linked, on hypochondria as well. Because, as it is an impasse in relational terms, possible equivalent of a somatization away from which projection keeps the subject, hypochondria calls forth Social and Biological for a complete overhaul of psychosis.

(2) For an explanatory definition providing hypochondria with a theoretical status; thanks to a different conceptual system, the main insights appear to be the following:

M. Derzelle, *Towards a Psychosomatic Conception of Hypochondria,*
DOI: 10.1007/978-3-319-03053-1_9,
© Springer International Publishing Switzerland 2014

- Belief in a mysteriously affected body including in its cipher a relationship to another person, hypochondria which is a projective process, failed repression whose proximity must be noticed with paranoia, is the development of a situation of impasse that reveals that a former character functioning turned into the prevalent adaptative attitude is inoperative.
- Impasse that has been overcome because it is embedded in the elaboration of the unthinkable, that is the impossible loss of the narcissistic object, on which the subject vitally depends, hypochondria needs to be situated in the context of Somatization, impassable impasse offered to thought in a typical symptomatic oscillation.
  Somatic first, it then becomes psychical, as the frequent succession, pointed in our examples, of allergy and hypochondriac bouts, as if the result-failure of the first triggered the beginning of psychosis.

(3) To the relational and/or transferential plan, hypochondria reveals two essential aspects and completes the weakening of the concept of Actual:

- Medically first, the objective impasse, linked to the fact that complaint is taken into account, should be read, it seems, as the repetition of a subjective impasse in terms of relationship, projective attempt of a restoration of a relationship to another person on the model of childhood. This relationship, in fact, is the repetition of an early relational situation, background constituent of body superego where the distortion of the maternal function, that equates "you must" with "you mustn't," prevents the subject from leaving the iterative field that holds him captive.
- Psychoanalytically, as it is an episode of failed repression between two repressions, that is a projective flash of occasional appearance, a sort of breach in a type of character functioning, hypochondria yet needs to be read as the memory of a highly iterative past. Because, if we reached Freud's conclusion that there is no transference where only a little Imaginary emerges, we would disregard that a single functioning against a single object is thus reiterated, across a life that seems absent to itself, with no possible change and until exhaustion: character transference which tirelessly transforms the other person into body superego, generated by repression and perpetuating it.

This last development deserves some explanations.

In the first place, giving transferential value to all forms of hypochondria, we consider that it is a second functioning linked to a first one in terms of inclusion: kind of parenthesis in parentheses, reaction of survival when, in critical moments, the Imaginary bursts in, to repeat a first projection. Because what is happening is not that a pathology is being overflown by another which absorbs it. Passing to the limit, staking one's all, hypochondria is the very last resort to avoid death and it projectively takes over from the character functioning "of before," partly lifting the ban on projection by a projection of the prohibition to project. Everything happens as if body superego, old transformation of the maternal object into an instance filling a relational void, was re-projected to question, through its loss, the subject and his feeling of being. This means that the transference specific to hypochondria extends the one of successful repression, provided that, however, we do not ignore that transference exists in one case whereas in the other it is, in the therapeutic situation, constantly transformed into superego instance. Successful repression or hypochondria: same functioning against the same object.

The legitimacy of this reduction implies solving a problem upstream: that of the essential link of character repression with the relational level, link constantly denied in the Freudian system which considers the Actual functioning as a "deficient functioning." How then can we define this typical relationship that is always created, automatically, taking no account of the real qualities of the other person which very quickly appears to be allocated the systematic role of body superego? What name can we give to this unique relationship to oneself and to the other person, fixed once for all in a character functioning intended to deny Difference to produce Identity? If this singularity which suggests a great complexity is ignored, transference seems absent in a situation devoid of the imaginary dimension. That is why character transference which reproduces a strange relationship to the other person, relationship of dependence and even of obedience, as if to the ordinary functioning was substituted a special functioning, taken in charge by the other person on the projective mode, in an imaginary complementarity.

Presupposition of any analytical work and epistemological gap violation intended to go beyond the psychoneurotic scope, transference, far from being an isolated set of affects or conducts, is indeed a structured set, an internalized unconscious *situation*, and finally appears to be the concept sought to extend analyzability. It must not be confused with projection that yet is part of it. It allows a definition of the body, of its symptoms, in terms of transferential function made of the possible repetitions consistent with various fixation points, referring to the constitution of functions as well as to those already established. This demonstrates how thinking hypochondria seems in fact inseparable from a conception of the subject as a totality known as psychosomatic and within which points of fixation of different levels can coexist, the "actual" or "neurotic" events then always taking place in a relation to the other person. This totality, sometimes can be identified from the beginning. This is the case for example here for Mrs. V.

A hypochondriac symptom can be part of a symptomatic complex, associating a cancerous somatization in the form of a non-metastatic relapse with the specific traits of a hystero-phobic (Sami-Ali 1987, p.126) character; this surely shatters the Freudian conceptual framework. Burst and overflow of a reference framework which cannot allow to conceive the coexistence, or at least the alternation, within the same subject, of several somatizations of different levels, i.e. the levels of Real Body and Imaginary Body considered in their dialectical opposition. Therefore, we need a thought seizing in its unity a stratification of symptoms whose variability in time has to be incorporated into a totality linked to a type of functioning.

Conception of a totality which the case of Mrs. V. invites to develop since we can observe in it, assembled into a combination of symptoms at the same distance between "pure" organicity and "pure" neurosis, three different formations respectively corresponding to three different states, different in their degree but not in their nature, of a same basal process: projective activity. Thus coexist in her, for a specific period and at various levels, the three following sets, predominant in turn:

- A hystero-phobic (Sami-Ali 1987, p.126) level where projection is at work, through a movement making it possible to return to the pleasure principle, typically accompanied by a spatial structuration exclusively controlled by a unique relation of reciprocal inclusions. Regression which operates on the transferential level, reviving a maternal figure on the other person, as well as on the level of fantasy with confinement phobias where the relation between "outside" and "inside" is reversed, and which allows to solve, in a very peculiar way, the Oedipus in a unique relationship where the other person, active or passive, is a narcissistic double.

- A hypochondriacal level, where the outline of a projection intended to create, inside a space devoid of depth, an unthinkable distance, over determines a pain that primitively reveals that distance could not be created using projection. If, as the associated thermal changes, headaches indicate that Mrs. V. has to suffer constantly in strict obedience to a sadistic figure (dependence), their time of onset in fact equally reveals the attempt to create a distance in the form of a tension (independence). In fact, the "migraine feeling" has a single function, perfectly identifiable: whether it comes as the final stop to an experience of pleasure, as a total blockage to the utterance of a desire or as the punishment for any active position, it breaks an otherness while pointing at its attempt. Paradox of a symptom combining opposite directions: obedience and desire to live.

- A "real" somatic level, where the failure of projection, indissolubly linked to the emergence of an always denied difference that suddenly, however, appears, without being this time once again reduced to identity, and is allied in our patient with a severe regression which, in her case, takes the form of a cancerization. Faced to what, for her, is completely unthinkable, i.e. inelaborable, or even unintegrable, to be and not to be different from her sister (figure of the mother, moreover), sister against whom she allowed herself one day to verbally express all her aggressiveness, Mrs. V. seemed to have no other possible remedy than a somatization affecting the Real Body, only way to "negotiate" what was conflicting and had just taken by surprise her relational system. Contradiction appears where there is an implicit logic of being which is that of identity: in the absence of an acceptance involving a change of thought structure which would allow to incorporate it (psychosis), only the biological and immunological level seems to be able to restore a relationship to another person momentarily interrupted by a projective fiasco that revealed its strangeness. In cancer here, immune evasion precisely inhibits the release of tumor antigens, with either site specific or central mechanisms. Pointing to an alternative that therefore reveals the biological value (Villemain 1989) of projective activity.

From projection at work to its failure, a continuum appears, crossed by a single line that irresistibly draws a permanent relational mode of extreme proximity to the other person linked to a specific space where distance is abolished. As difference is inconceivable to a subject deprived of any possibility to exist except in the other person, the symptomatic changes, all of which have this common point to posit the individual as unique, are therefore the avatars of a same basic functioning. On this background projective continuum, a sort of barycenter, of balance point, stands out, as an average, or constant at least, functioning: hypochondriac symptoms, where the head, transit point between inside and outside, is without doubt the most invested part of the body. Migraines and thermal changes of the skull and top of the face indeed constantly emerge, greatly scaring Mrs. V., for whom this region is the object of major concern. What should be added, without putting aside the possibility of an overdetermination of symptoms, is that the problem in this case, more than location, is pain, pain with no end, synonymous with dependence and therefore of lack of distance: the impossibility of a pleasure which would be independence and even disobedience derives therefrom.

The problem of Mrs. V., as it appears in therapy, is thus entirely centered on the search for a personal identity, that has been supplanted until then by the unyielding will of being one with the mother, and intensified by sexual identity, once we have interpreted the anal sexual language (strong/weak) which absorbs the patient by preventing her from existing in any way but as a mother experienced in her omnipotence to which she had always tried to identify. Her questioning in the form of a "who am I?" quickly followed by a "when am I me?" is from this point of view instructive, which directs her existence around a dependence to another person who controls the temporal dimension for her (Sami-Ali 1990, pp.69–104). In any other language, borrowed to D. Anzieu, Mrs. V. is dependent on an impossible border:

> uncertainties on the borders between Psychic Ego and Body Ego, between Reality-Ego and Ego-Ideal, between what depends on oneself and what depends on others, abrupt fluctuations of these borders, accompanied by descents into depression, undifferentiation of erogenous zones, confusion of pleasurable and painful experiences, instinctual indistinction because of which the rise of a drive is felt as violence and not as desire, vulnerability to narcissistic injury due to the weakness or faults in the psychic envelope, diffuse feeling of malaise, feeling of not living one's own life, of seeing one's body and thoughts operate from the outside, of being the spectator of something that is and that is not one's own existence (Anzieu 1985).

All those states need to be organized around two main axes: considering the double level of the problem, as much Oedipal (gender identity) as essentially dual (personal identity), their combined study is required. To Freud's diachronic model we therefore prefer the synchronic one, engaging the subject in a problem that at the same time, pertains to several levels.

Mrs. V. is 56 but "confesses" it difficultly; she owns a big *bar-tabac*[*]. Typical family business where she has worked for a long time with her husband and her two sons to whom, with difficulties, she is gradually handing over, since a breast cancer has made her permanently tired. In her decision to start a psychotherapy, what prevails is somatic complaint on analgesic-resistant cephalalgias that have become her companions in life. With no identifiable rhythmicity or significant triggering factor, they are a sort of constant background and seem in charge of constituting the unity, or even the continuity of her existence. Against this background, there are paroxystic, painful violent migraine crises. As pain increases, vision is blurred, and all activities involving first and foremost "sight" must be canceled: reading for example is impossible. The first crisis was sometimes mentioned as perhaps dating back to when her mother beat her to punish her for having stolen flowers from the cemetery, as she was 8 years old. Mrs. V. remembers the sudden pain gripped her "like a gunshot," across the head and confined her to bed. For her, the prohibition to retort, the inability to express feelings, keystones of her education, are the explanations of this headache to which she assigns a meaning of retention at the same time as one of a rumination. "Shut up and endure do not prevent from thinking," but then distance is disobedience, that the painful crisis seems to punish.

In addition to these headaches a depression then consumes her life. Another dimension highlighted during a consultation mainly centered on pain and which first had a medical framework; we meet her for the first time, with a doctor she has already seen, to whom she has just said that she could not take it anymore (This patient was initially seen in the context of the Pain Management Consultation that we provide with Dr. Christian Pozzo di Borgo, head of the Department of Anaesthesia and Intensive Care at the Institut Jean Godinot (Reims)).

Crying, Mrs. V. narrates her difficulties, chaotic and tangled words where the word "uselessness" emerges repeatedly.

- Uselessness of drugs whose action only lasts a moment, thus resulting in excesses in which quantity has nothing to do with comfort. Moreover, Mrs. V., in total despair, confesses her project of throwing everything away.
- Uselessness of her horizon, in which the prospect of a retirement, become "necessary" not because of her age but due to a desire to "have things settled" which has been constant since "you-know-what," is probably the biggest cloud. Mrs. V. finds herself stuck in a process she has initiated: wishing to make an *inter-vivos* gift recommended to her by all her entourage and which would allow her to retire, she cannot think of stopping "work," when she imagines her future days all alike and empty. This ambivalence leads her to deny what she expressed only a few moments before: her weakened resistance, her fatigability. If it turns out that "working," for her, is existing, why survive if it were to stop?
- Uselessness of her existence, whose meaning she questions at the time of a highly negative assessment exacerbated by her depressive background and that refers her to the difficult mourning of a grandiose, ideal, self-image. Because what really has to be reconsidered because of an adaptation related to cancer and its aftermath, seems Mrs. V.'s apparent organization of her relational mode. Stopping her activity is the threat of a real danger that is, for her, of existential nature: the vital and constant identification with a figure experienced as an all-powerful, maternal figure whose requirements forbid any sort of difference. Mrs. V. has to work, otherwise she will lose her identity. This reveals the paradox of existing avoiding to be different from the other, to suppress oneself in order to exist, in short to be a subject by the very movement where subjectivity is annihilated.

The initial phase of therapy shows that depression here means a work of mourning almost impossible to begin, extreme resistance to a process of extrication from the Similar—which we think should be named disidentification. More than migraines, it immediately occupies a very concerned center stage. Mrs. V. has to make a major change which endangers an identity whose illusion consists in nondistance, revealed inter alia by her headaches. If the prospect of difference causes, as such, a depression, it therefore means that the issue is important, and we unambiguously locate it on the side of an identity disorder: risk of depersonalization (how to be both the other person and the other's other) and risk of annihilation (being nothing if one is not the other) thus alternate during therapy, in a swinging alternation of "all or nothingness," on the Oedipal level as on the dual level.

To closely report, in their emergence and their movement, the different levels of a problem whose first feature is a symptomatic variability where somatic forms prevail, we have chosen, exceptionally, to note as such or in summary, what was said during two sessions. They took place approximately 6 months after the first face-to-face sessions which were totally devoted to somatic complaint and to a description of current facts, with no mention of any story.

It is on the basis of a dream which reflects the precise meaning of transferential evolution that Mrs. V. finally accepts to speak about herself. "I had a funny dream last night, and you were there." I was in a kind of coma on the sidewalk, out in the street. A thought obsessed me and came to my mind repeatedly: "Nobody will come pick me up." My mother was there, indifferent. My whole family was there, indifferent. I saw them watching me suffer, without reaction. My husband was painting, as usual. A neighbor, whose face I could not see, took me under the arm and dragged me in a house, well, no, it was a garage. It was awful, this state of discomfort, on the ground, unconscious. I could not move and I told myself: "I'm still nothing. Nobody is interested in me." And then I recognized you: the neighbor, it was you." And adopting an interpretation previously given in which headache had the meaning of "being like" the mother, she tells me that she thought upon awakening that salvation came therefore to her from the Stranger (me) instead of the Familiar (relatives).

In this dream filled with transferential information, two points are directly particularly meaningful:

- On the one hand, the figuration of the analytical sofa-chair arrangement where the patient is reclining, so that motricity ("a kind of coma," "I could not move") as well as vision ("a neighbor whose face I could not see") are put out of action, inviting to favor verbal and auditory activity, is the prefiguration of the future situation, presented as a perspective of speakability: it can be interpreted as a request for analysis, for coming closer to allow the investigation to begin. The distance that Mrs. V. created in not opening up is ultimately only a defense against a positive transference in formation. Evidenced, if need be, by the role of the neighbor that she assigns to me: her salvation only depends on me, salvation that is being saved from death represented as a denarcissization ("I am still nothing. No one is interested in me.").

- On the other hand, we can notice that the theme of the face (Sami-Ali 1977, pp.117–150), carried by a typical transferential process tending to move from the disinvestment of familiar faces (the mother's face to which the family is reduced) to the final investment of a recognized stranger's face (implying that it must first be known as and therefore perceived as different), raises demand for analysis as a quest for an identity. Such is Mrs. V.'s essential issue: breaking the reciprocity in the exchanges with the familiar ("I saw them watch me suffer, without reaction"), maintaining no more the constitutive illusion of a first identity (having the mother's face), the loss that coma expresses is the one of self-identity as a face. Loss symbolized here by the narcissistic double represented by the neighbor whose unperceived face, not visible from the point of view of the other person, is a risk of annihilation: enigma of the subject without face and promise of the face.

Program-dream, therefore, this inaugural dream can be read in spatial or temporal terms, two complementary aspects united in transference. Oneiric activity thus heralds the change in the latter. A second session recorded about three months later exemplarily confirms this as it repeats with the analyst, on the transferential level, a relationship to the other person as body superego: evocation by Mrs. V. of her depression, her problems, of the perspective of her upcoming retirement which, for the first time, occupy the foreground, relegating to second place the migraines that she hardly speaks of at the end of the session. This makes her nasty, aggressive: the row with her husband in the morning shows it. She says she takes everything the wrong way and feels rejected. She who, boss lady, has always given a lot, has supported the others in many occasions, is disappointed not be supported by anybody now that she needs it. Her activity has often led her to receive misfits, people with problems, and now, her sons have sent her home "like a grandmother." Feels useless.... Even her children do not understand.... She feels rejected.... The two younger sons who work with her have even told her to come to the Balmoral (name of her bar) only if she feels like it, and to take time for self-care instead. Take care of herself! Mrs. V. has never done it, has never felt the need to do it. Today, she was expecting a warm welcome with another son of hers: he wasn't even there! "I should not have gone, I would have avoided a disappointment."

She talks about important relationship problems with her husband, but this is not recent. She has difficulties to say what occupies his mind: a tension and a kind of weariness. "He is a man of the past," and by that she means "who remains attached to past stories." Married this man when she was 17 years old and he was 26: "I was much too young." This marriage is described as a marriage of convenience, "without love and without passion." With respect to the sexual act, Mrs. V. insists on the repugnance it has always inspired her.... Think about sexuality.... Of course, she has never refused anything to her husband but has always kept her indifference quiet. "Pleasure, never experienced." A certain time after their marriage, returned from deportation, Mr. V. went to Belgium for 4 years to work as an auto-body mechanic, his first profession. Mrs. V. remained in France, occupied to set up a laundry business with one of her sisters: it was her who chose not to go with her husband. During his absence, she had "overnight adventures." *Wonder what I'll be thinking of her…. Expects to be scolded, even slapped….* Oscillates between an attempt to justify herself: "I'm human," and a major guilt: it was a deception… a sin… she should not have done it…. "And, I'm a believer" she repeats insistently, *using religion as a model of compliance as well as the prohibition of any pleasure.* Also wonders if she does not refrain "from inside" all sorts of pleasure using the "exterior" backing of religion.

Thinks about when her jealous husband returned from Belgium…. This topic, she wants to avoid it…. This image, especially…. A force obliges her not to talk about it… and to dismiss the vision that is coming…. The bedroom…. A stop…. Her thoughts take her back, as if it was yesterday, to the scene so many times repeated: she sees her husband, obsessed with the idea of what could have happened during his absence, wake her up in the middle of night to question her, clutching her neck…. Feels his hands strangling her…. She's afraid…. The past merges with the present and remembrance acquires an almost sensory materiality. It is this oppressive, too strong, presence that Mrs. V. is unable to stand. Oppression felt each time that her husband came up with this old story, questioning her for confession…. Recalls when, in her childhood, her mother beat her…. Again, the image of the bedroom…. Mrs. V. strives not to think about this scene and tries to turn away from this unbearable representation. Her mind is confused…. (*A headache has just begun!*) Pain helps avoiding the situation. Can no longer speak, doesn't think anything. "What you think of me?" "I am good for nothing." What she is sure of, is that her husband loves her. As evidenced by his jealousy. Certainly, at the time she considered a separation because he terrorized her so much but, in the words of her mother, "in the family, nobody divorces." Very quickly pregnant with her first child, she left marital home shortly after birth to come back a few weeks later because, in the words of her mother again, "this child needed a father" (*Headache goes on*).

Her life seemed wasted: no passion, no real intimate life, but reason, duty, work. Images dating from the past: her mother who worked hard, whom she had never seen inactive and who transmitted the sense of family to her…. Thinks of a possible success of her own existence as a mother…. She has four sons, who have given her twelve grandchildren…. Immediately dismisses this idea…. She doubts…. Her sons have made their way: the eldest is an engineer, the second an automotive expert, the last two work in the bar, but none understands her. All this has led to nothing…. Mrs. V. hypothesizes that they did not perceive the internal change of their mother, as that they are prisoners of their need to keep the image of a strong woman. Her husband shares this point of view. Worst of all, he believes she is faking! Moreover, it was always her who "wore the breeches" in business: bank, papers, management, etc. Her husband would have been unable to manage all this, and he is indeed uncomfortable with the idea. He needs her, would be nothing without her, perhaps a bum…. Is this not her yet who initiated their business success, for having decided their job change one morning? Do away with laundry and auto-body! The idea proved good, even if the initial debt lead M. V. to depression.... Mrs. V. supported him with all her strength. However, how much she would have liked, for a husband, to have a strong and solid man to support her! Daydreaming (*Headache*). This pulls toward passivity, but she wants to leave this state, she refuses to remain silent, in a passive position toward me.

Returns to what she already said at the beginning of the session: the fear of retirement.... Doing nothing, getting bored: this is not possible.... She has to do something... to be active.... Work, that's her specialty! Associates ideas about her childhood, dominated by the figure of a very hard mother who made her start to work at the age of 13. In the family there were two older sisters and two twins, younger half-brothers born to the mother's second marriage. The father of Mrs. V. died when she was 2 years old, of a fall. She doesn't remember him.... On the contrary, remembers very well she was interested in studies, she would have liked to continue despite maternal opposition but with the encouragement of a teacher who understood her and helped a lot.... Even though she could have benefited from scholarships which would have solved the financial problem, her mother did not give up: "Work in the factory, you'll earn money, and right away!" At the age of 13, Mrs. V. therefore found herself in a glass factory, striving to provide the best possible performance in order to get paid more and bring more money to her mother (up to 42 cents a day instead of 24 as planned). Work... and so that it pays off.... Did what her mother told her to do, although she did not want to.... "Work, yes, but not for myself." This memory awakens the image of the pocket change that was left to her for her hairdresser, her makeup, her stockings.... Her mother appears to her, in counter-point, as the woman who had "all" while she had "nothing".... She felt weak, small, in her presence.... For her she embodied authority.... She sees her, as if she were there, giving orders, hiring each of her children to specific tasks she distributed to them.... Laundry, dishes, wall-paper.... Admiration rises: "She could build walls by herself!" (*Remains speechless, taking her head between her hands*). "Being nothing".... This sensation affects the relationship that Mrs. V. has with me: the same image of my superiority and consequently of her inferiority invades everything....

Envy.... Envy for this mother "both male and female. She was both parents at the same time".... The feeling of inferiority or need for another person that she could consider as superior therefore covers the wish to be man and woman at a time, illusion of a possible omnipotence proceeding from the negation of the difference of sexes, the difference between father and mother. His father... She does not know much about him.... He was a stone sculptor and, as an artist should, left nothing to his wife and children.... The past takes her back to the present: Mrs. V. is bothered by the *inter vivos* gift that she would like to give her children, but that separates them into two clans. Not to be like her father... but like her mother.... Role of money in the family strife.... Does not understand why the older sons do not agree: the proposed sum as a compensation for the assets of the younger sons seems to be fair. There is a link between this case and her own story: the difference in treatment between her and her two sisters whom she envied, was

jealous of.... Her mother preferred them.... She received the blows, the thrash-
ings.... No longer wants to think about it. *Wonders what she has in her head to feel*
such a pain. Fear of losing her head. "Confesses" having deliberately committed
some petty theft to attract maternal wrath on her.... Considers that it was evil from
the point of view of religion.... Went to confession.... Always feels at fault.... She
wonders why she suddenly thinks of her mother's second marriage, "by convenience," to ensure the financial security of the family. By convenience....

Me—By convenience?

Her—Yes, as I did myself, as if my life had to reproduce that of my mother.

Me—Had to?

Mrs. V. is silent then, speaking slowly, in a low voice interspersed with silences
reflecting a change of level in associative speech, says this is stunning, providing
the interpretation herself: she has always lived as if she had internalized her
mother's orders, continues to follow them as if she was still there. Pride on her
part? Love instead, desire to be like her. Associates ideas on the similarities
between the parental couple and hers. Was surprised to discover all the things that
confirm them: work, make money, strong woman image. The mourning of the
ideal image of herself that she has to go through is above all the one of a relationship with the mother.

But there is something else.... Thinks of her two breast cancers.... Impression that
these events which happened 3 years ago are now lost in the mists of time.... Feeling
that all this has slid off her back.... Nothing significant, nothing traumatic.... Critical
of the attitude of media about cancer.... Everything happened very quickly....
Remembers the chronology of her double illness.... Her first tumor in the right breast
was operated in a private surgery, with no axillary lymph node dissection. It was a
mistake. It proved necessary shortly later. Memories of radiotherapy sessions....
Discovery, the following year of a tumor in the left breast, much smaller. Another
operation. Feels like saying that all this had no effect on her.... For her sex life, she
asked her husband not to touch this area, through modesty, but also because of the
painful aftermath. Three years already! Implies the representation of a splitting
which helped her withstand the rays. She thought: "Only my body is here, I am
somewhere else".... Her mother, by the way....

Me—What is the relation between cancer and your mother?

Just remembers that her mother died of uterine cancer.... Significant bleeding
about which, as she was more than 80, she had refused to see a doctor, calling them
"periods return".... Admiration for this strong mother who refused to seek
treatment.... She had worked until the age of seventy before devoting herself, ideal
grandmother, to her grandchildren. Mrs. V.'s children kept a very good image of
her.... Realizes that her image of her mother is different from theirs.... Ah yes!
Migraine headaches! "It's the maternal side." Mrs. V.'s grandmother and mother
have had them all their lives long.... Her mother had even predicted a decrease
around menopause.... And it happened: 2 years of tranquility.... Otherwise, she
thinks she has always suffered from them, with violent crises at the time of her
menstruation, in general very painful, and, as a teenager, when she felt upset, often

in connection with unspoken conflicts with her mother.... Effects of the word of maternal lineage on the body....

Asks me, before leaving, whether it is necessary for her to go to the Balmoral or not today.

Me—Why, if it is necessary?

Her—It's always the same thing! I don't know what to do anymore.... It was clear before....

Me—Before? Before what?

Her—Before my illness. When I could do everything.

Cries and has trouble leaving. "Leaving is always difficult, but as my mother used to say, everything has an end."

No doubt this session can be subsumed under the central concept of body superego. Major guideline present on several levels that reveal a personality organization which oscillates through time between cancer and psychosis as equivalents; in fact, it means a relational mode where the subject, to avoid being a separate term, is continuously united with requirements that violate her, certainly, but give her existence. They have successively the face of the mother, of morality or religion, they seek mine even within transference, but they just repeat a first projection. If this proximity just happens to disappear, loss of self-esteem by the loss of the object that is self, projection recreates another person on the imaginary level to fill the gap as formerly. Thus hypochondria is a deployment of a wider symptomatic variability, comprehensive and psychosomatic process where "psychic" alternates with "somatic," whose continuity ultimately tell a single functioning against a single object.

9.1 As a Conclusion

Thought, and Freud's throughout his life, as well as his work vividly revealed it, is a distance, a point of balance around the hole, a gap maintained between what fills and what digs, marriage renewed with the unknown, fantastic desire of what you cannot regain. As Montaigne says:

> Even if we let our thoughts cut and sew to their pleasure, they cannot even desire what is proper to them and so be satisfied (Montaigne 1588).

Distance, gap, mark and limit. Thought has the protective power of skin. The elaboration of this work was undoubtedly involved in the defense and constitution of ours.

> Don't take this symptom away from me, I need it more than my life, do not take me this thought on which I formed an identity—fragile, debt-ridden—but an identity (Schneider 1982).

Our own thought, essential symptom.

References

Abraham K (1966) Développement de la libido. In: Œuvres complètes, tome II. Payot, Paris

Abraham N, Torok M (1978) L'écorce et le noyau. Aubier-Flammarion, Paris. English edition: Abraham N, Torok M (1994) The shell and the kernel: renewals of psychoanalysis. University of Chicago Press, Chicago

Alexander F (1965) Psychosomatic medicine: its principles and applications. Norton, New York

Anzieu D (1985) Le Moi-peau. Dunod, Paris

Aulagnier P (1987) Les destins du plaisir. Dunod, Paris

Bachelard G (1947) L'eau et les rêves. José Corti, Paris

Bailly A (1950) Dictionnaire grec-français. Hachette, Paris

Balint M (1967) The basic fault (2nd edn, 1984). Routledge, London

Baumeyer F (1955) The Schreber case. Int J Psychoanal 37(1):61–74. French edition: Baumeyer F (1979) Le cas Schreber. In: Le cas Schreber. P.U.F., Paris

Calligaris C (1987) Que veut l'hypochondriaque? Ornicar. no. 14

Celerier MC (1978) De la causalité psychosomatique. In: Topique, Epi. dec. 1978, no. 22

Clavreul J (1978) L'ordre médical. Seuil, Paris

Codet H (1939) Les deux hypocondries. Mélanges offerts à P. Janet. D'Artrey, Paris

Cotard J (1891) Étude sur les maladies cérébrales et mentales. Baillière, Paris

Cottraux J (1976) L'hypocondriaque et le médecin imaginaire ou le corps médical face au corps malade. In: Psychothérapies médicales. Tome II. Masson, Paris

Delahousse J, Hitter-Spinelli B (1980) Discours hypocondriaque et discours médical. In: Revue de Médecine Psychosomatique, 22 no. 1

Derzelle E, Gorot J (1991) L'investigation psychosomatique en gastro-entérologie. Technique et intérêt. In: Mignon M (ed) Précis de Gastroentérologie. Ellipses, Paris

Durandeaux J (1982) Poétique analytique. Seuil, Paris

Ey H (1950) Étude no. 17: l'hypocondrie. In: Etudes Psychiatriques, Tome II. Desclée de Brouwer, Paris

Fedida P (1971) L'anatomie dans la psychanalyse. In: Nouvelle Revue de Psychanalyse, 3

Fedida P (1975) Une plainte restée en souffrance. Psychologie Médicale 7(4)

Fedida P (1977a) A propos du somatique. In: Corps du vide et espace de séance. Jean-Pierre Delarge, Paris

Fedida P (1977b) L'hypochondrie du rêve. In: Corps du vide et espace de séance. Jean-Pierre Delarge, Paris

Fedida P (1978a) La théorie somatique dans la psychanalyse. Psychanalyse à l'université Réplique, vol 3, no. 12

Fedida P (1978b) L'absence. Gallimard, Paris

Fenichel O (1946) The psychoanalytic theory of neurosis. Kegan Paul, Trench, Trubner, London

Ferenczi S (1919) English edition: Ferenczi S (1969) The psycho-analysis of a case of hysterical hypochondria. In: Further contributions to the theory and technique of psychoanalysis. Hogarth Press, London

Ferenczi S (1922) English edition: Ferenczi S (1955) Psychoanalysis and the mental disorders of general paralysis. In: Further contributions to the problems and methods of psychoanalysis. Hogarth Press, London

Ferenczi S (1932) French edition: Ferenczi S (1985) Journal clinique. Payot, Paris

Feyerabend P (1975) Against method. New Left Books, New York. French edition: Feyerabend P (1979) Contre la méthode. Seuil, Paris

Ford C (1983) The somatizing disorders. Elsevier Biomedical, New York

Foucault M (1966) Les mots et les choses. Gallimard, Paris

Freud A (1957) Le rôle de la maladie somatique dans la vie psychique des enfants. Revue Française de Psychanalyse, 21 no. 5

Freud S (1887–1904) Extracts from the Fliess papers. Draft B. In: Freud S (1966) The standard edition of the complete psychological works of Sigmund Freud, vol 1 (trans: Strachey J (ed)). Hogarth Press, London

Freud S (1892–1895) Studies on Hysteria. In: Freud S (1955) The standard edition of the complete psychological works of Sigmund Freud, vol 2 (trans: Strachey J (ed)). Hogarth Press, London

Freud S (1894) Qu'il est justifié de séparer de la neurasthénie un certain complexe symptomatique sous le nom de névrose d'angoisse. In: Freud S (1973) Névrose, psychose et perversion. French edition: (trans: Laplanche J (ed)). P.U.F., Paris

Freud S (1904 [1903]) Freud's psychoanalytical procedure. In: Freud S (1953) The standard edition of the complete psychological works of Sigmund Freud, vol 7 (trans: Strachey J (ed)). Hogarth Press, London

Freud S (1908) On the sexual theories of children. In: Freud S (1959) The standard edition of the complete psychological works of Sigmund Freud, vol 9 (trans: Strachey J (ed)). Hogarth Press, London

Freud S (1911) Psychoanalytical notes on an autobiographical account of a case of Paranoia. In: Freud S (1958) The standard edition of the complete psychological works of Sigmund Freud, vol 12 (trans: Strachey J (ed)). Hogarth Press, London

Freud S (1912–1913) Totem and Taboo. In: Freud S (1955) The standard edition of the complete psychological works of Sigmund Freud, vol 13 (trans: Strachey J (ed)). Hogarth Press, London

Freud S (1914) On Narcissism: an introduction. In: Freud S (1957) The standard edition of the complete psychological works of Sigmund Freud, vol 14 (trans: Strachey J (ed)). Hogarth Press, London

Freud S (1915) The unconscious. In: Freud S (1957) The standard edition of the complete psychological works of Sigmund Freud, vol 14 (trans: Strachey J (ed)). Hogarth Press, London

Freud S (1915 [1917]a) A metapsychological supplement to the theory of dreams. In: Freud S (1957) The standard edition of the complete psychological works of Sigmund Freud, vol 14 (trans: Strachey J (ed)). Hogarth Press, London

Freud S (1915 [1917]b) Mourning and Melancholia. In: Freud S (1957) The standard edition of the complete psychological works of Sigmund Freud, vol 14 (trans: Strachey J (ed)). Hogarth Press, London

Freud S (1915–1916) Introductory lectures on psycho-analysis. In: Freud S (1963) The standard edition of the complete psychological works of Sigmund Freud, vol 15 (trans: Strachey J (ed)). Hogarth Press, London

Freud S (1916–1917) Introductory lectures on psycho-analysis. In: Freud S (1963) The standard edition of the complete psychological works of Sigmund Freud, vol 16 (trans: Strachey J (ed)). Hogarth Press, London

Freud S (1919) The uncanny. In: Freud S (1955) The standard edition of the complete psychological works of Sigmund Freud, vol 17 (trans: Strachey J (ed)). Hogarth Press, London

Freud S (1921) Group psychology and the analysis of the ego. In: Freud S (1955) The standard edition of the complete psychological works of Sigmund Freud, vol 18 (trans: Strachey J (ed)). Hogarth Press, London

Freud S (1924) The economic problem of Masochism. In: Freud S (1961) The standard edition of the complete psychological works of Sigmund Freud, vol 19 (trans: Strachey J (ed)). Hogarth Press, London

Freud S (1925) Inhibitions, symptoms and anxiety. In: Freud S (1955) The standard edition of the complete psychological works of Sigmund Freud, vol 20 (trans: Strachey J (ed)). Hogarth Press, London

Freud S (1937) Analysis terminable and interminable. In: Freud S (1964) The standard edition of the complete psychological works of Sigmund Freud, vol 23 (trans: Strachey J (ed)). Hogarth Press, London

Freud S (1939) Moses and Monotheism: Three essays. In: Freud S (1964) The standard edition of the complete psychological works of Sigmund Freud, vol 23 (trans: Strachey J (ed)). Hogarth Press, London

Freud S (1956) Lettre no. 17 du 19-04-1894. In: La naissance de la psychanalyse. P.U.F., Paris

Freud S (1973a) Introduction à la psychanalyse. Payot, Paris

Freud S (1973b) Qu'il est justifié de séparer de la neurasthénie un certain complexe symptomatique sous le nom de "névrose d'angoisse". In: Névrose, psychose et perversion (trans: Laplanche J (ed)). P.U.F., Paris

Freud S (1984) Sigmund Freud présenté par lui-même. Gallimard, Paris

Greenfield N, Roessler R (1958) Hypochondria: a new conception of the problem. J Ment Dis 126(5)

Igoin L (1979) La boulimie et son infortune. P.U.F, Paris

Jones E (1955) Sigmund Freud, life and work II. Hogarth Press, London

Kenyon FE (1966) Hypochondriasis: a survey of some historical, clinical and social aspects. Int J Psychiatry 2(3):301–334

Kenyon FE (1976) Hypochondrial states. Br J Psychiatry 129

Klein M (1940) Mourning and its relation to manic-depressive states. In: Klein M (1986) The selected Melanie Klein. Hogarth Press, London

Klein M (1935) A contribution to the psychogenesis of manic-depressive states. In: Klein M (1986) The selected Melanie Klein. Hogarth Press, London

Klein M (1968) Essais de psychanalyse. Payot, Paris

Lacan J (1932) De la psychose paranoïaque dans ses rapports avec la personnalité. Le François, Paris

Laplanche J, Pontalis JB (1967) Vocabulaire de la psychanalyse. P.U.F., Paris

Lebovici S (1969) Indications et contre-indications de la psychanalyse freudienne. In: Encyclopédie Médico-Chirurgicale, Psychiatrie, III, 37811, A 10, 5, 7

Magnan V, Serieux P (1890) Le délire chronique à évolution systématique. Masson, Paris

Marty P (1980) L'ordre psychosomatique. Payot, Paris

Maurel H (1973) Actualité de l'hypocondrie. In: Rapport de psychiatrie au 73ème congrès de psychiatrie et de neurologie de langue française. Masson, Paris

McDougall J (1980) Plea for a measure of abnormality. International Universities Press, New York

McDougall J (1982) Théâtres du Je. Gallimard, Paris

McDougall J (1985) Theaters of the mind. Harper Collins, New York

Montaigne M (1588) Les Essais

Nunberg H (1932) Allgemeine Neurosenlehre auf psychoanalytischer Grundlage. Huber, Bern

Perrier F (1978) Psychanalyse de l'hypocondriaque. In: La chaussée d'Antin-Antienne. 10/18, Paris

Pontalis JB (1977) Entre le rêve et la douleur. Gallimard, Paris

Rosolato G (1978) La relation d'inconnu. Gallimard, Paris

Roustang F (1970) Influence. Éditions de Minuit, Paris

Roustang F (1976) Un destin si funeste. Editions de Minuit, Paris

Sami-Ali M (1970) De la projection. Une étude psychanalytique. Payot, Paris

Sami-Ali M (1974) La convergence visuelle: In: L'espace imaginaire. Gallimard, Paris

Sami-Ali M (1977) Corps réel, corps imaginaire. Dunod, Paris

Sami-Ali M (1980) Le banal. Gallimard, Paris

Sami-Ali M (1982) Penser le somatique. Nouvelle revue de psychanalyse, 25

Sami-Ali M (1984) Le visuel et le tactile. Essai sur la psychose et l'allergie. Dunod, Paris

Sami-Ali M (1987) Penser le somatique. Imaginaire et pathologie. Dunod, Paris

Sami-Ali M (1990) Le corps, l'espace et le temps. Dunod, Paris

Sapir M (1980) Soignant-soigné : le corps à corps. Payot, Paris

Schilder P (1935) The image and appearance of the human body. Kegan Paul, Trench, Trubner, London

Schneider M (1982) A quoi penses-tu ? Nouvelle Revue de Psychanalyse. 25

Schreber DP (1903) English edition: Schreber DP (1955) Memoirs of my nervous illness. President and Fellows of Harvard College. Cambridge

Sperling M (1978) Psychosomatic disorders in children. Jason Aronson, New York

Spitz R (1965) The first year of life. International University Press, New York

Tausk V (1933) On the origin of the influencing machine in schizophrenia. Psychoanal Q 2(4):519–556

Tort P (1983) La pensée hiérarchique et l'évolution. Aubier, Paris

Valabrega JP (1980) Phantasme, mythe, corps et sens. Payot, Paris, p 15

Villemain F (1989) Stress et immunologie. P.U.F., Paris

Further Readings

Abraham K (1966) Le pronostic du traitement psychanalytique chez les sujets d'un certain âge. In: Œuvres complètes. Tome II. Petite bibliothèque Payot, Paris

Ajuriaguerra J de, Tissot R (1977) Aspect psychologique de la sénescence. In: Abrégé de Gérontologie? Masson, Paris

Amado Levy-Valensi E (1965) Le temps dans la vie psychologique. Flammarion, Paris

Anzieu D (1974) Vers une métapsychologie de la création. In: Psychanalyse du génie créateur. Dunod, Paris

Anzieu D (1975) Le transfert paradoxal. Nouvelle Revue de Psychanalyse, 12

Balint M (1972) Les voies de la régression. French edition: (trans: Dupont J, Viliker M). Payot, Paris

Bercheree P (1983) Genèse des concepts freudiens. Navarin, Paris

Bergeret J (1974) La dépression et les états limites. Payot, Paris

Bernard M (1976) Le corps Corps et culture, Editions universitaires, Paris

Berthaux P (1972) Le vieillissement normal et pathologique. Revue du Praticien 22:2

Binswanger L (1970) Discours, parcours et Freud. French edition: (trans: Lewinter R). Gallimard, Paris

Busse EW, Dovenmuehle RH, Brown RG (1960) Psychoneurotic reactions of the aged. Geriatrics, 15

Canguilhem G (1966) Le normal et le pathologique. P.U.F., Paris

Canguilhem G (1975) La connaissance de la vie. Vrin, Paris

Cottraux J (1974) Narcissisme, pensée médicale et pensée psychotique. Evolution psychiatrique, 1

Cottraux J (1976) Discours hypocondriaque et discours médical ou l'esprit de corps. Psychologie médicale, 8(5):777–779

Cottraux J (1977) Paradoxe, agir et imaginaire corporel chez l'hypocondriaque. Evolution psychiatrique 42(2):729–735

Dedieu-Anglade G (1961) Contribution à l'étude des névroses d'involution. Dissertation, Paris

Dejours C (1986) Le corps entre biologie et psychanalyse. Payot, Paris

Delahousse J (1976) A la recherche d'un effet d'ouverture chez l'hypocondriaque. L'Encéphale, 2

Delahousse J, Couvez A (1973) L'hypocondrie ou le contenu explosif. In: Rapport du congrès de psychiatrie et neurologie de langue française, 73th session, pp 295–299 Masson, Paris

Dupre E, Camus P (1907) Les cénestopathies. Encéphale, 11

Ey H, Brisset C, Bernard P (1974) Les troubles mentaux de la sénilité. In: Manuel de psychiatrie. Masson, Paris

Ferenczi S (1917) Les pathonévroses. In: Œuvres complètes, Tome II. French edition: Ferenczi S (1968) (trans: Dupont J et al.). Payot, Paris

Ferenczi S (1921) Pour comprendre les psychonévroses du retour d'âge. In: Œuvres complètes, Tome III. French edition: Ferenczi S (1968) (trans: Dupont J and all). Payot, Paris

Foucault M (1961) Histoire de la folie à l'âge classique. Pion, Paris

M. Derzelle, *Towards a Psychosomatic Conception of Hypochondria*,
DOI: 10.1007/978-3-319-03053-1,
© Springer International Publishing Switzerland 2014

Foucault M (1963) Naissance de la clinique. P.U.F, Paris

Freud S (1805) Trois essais sur la théorie de la sexualité. French edition : Freud S (1962) (trans: Reverchon-Jouve B). Gallimard, Paris

Freud S (1894) Les psychonévroses de défense. In: Freud S (1973) Névrose, psychose et perversion (trans: Laplanche J). P.U.F., Paris

Freud S (1896) L'hérédité et l'étiologie des névroses. In: Freud S (1973) Névrose, psychose et perversion (trans: Laplanche J). P.U.F., Paris

Freud S (1896) Nouvelles remarques sur les psychonévroses de défense. In: Freud S (1973) Névrose, psychose et perversion (trans: Laplanche J). P.U.F., Paris

Freud S (1899) Sur les souvenirs écrans. In: Freud S (1973) Névrose, psychose et perversion (trans: Berger D, Bruno P, Guerineau D, Oppenot F). P.U.F., Paris

Freud S (1912) Sur les types d'entrée dans la névrose. In: Freud S (1973) Névrose, psychose et perversion (trans: Laplanche J). P.U.F., Paris

Freud S (1915) Le refoulement. In: Freud S (1968) Métapsychologie (trans: Laplanche J and Pontalis JB). Gallimard, Paris

Freud S (1915) Les pulsions et leur destin. In: Freud S (1968) Métapsychologie (trans: Laplanche J and Pontalis JB). Gallimard, Paris

Freud S (1924) Névrose et psychose. In: Freud S (1973) Névrose, psychose et perversion (trans: Laplanche J). P.U.F., Paris

Freud S, Andreas Salome L (1912–1936) Correspondance. French edition: Freud S, Andreas Salome L (1970) (trans: Jumel L). Gallimard, Paris

Freud S, Pfister O (1909–1939) Correspondance. French edition: Freud S, Pfister O (1966) (trans: Jumel L). Gallimard, Paris

Gantheret F (1971) Remarques sur la place et le statut du corps en psychanalyse. Nouvelle Revue de Psychanalyse, 3

Green A (1974) L'analyste, la symbolisation et l'absence dans le cadre analytique. Nouvelle Revue de Psychanalyse, 10

Green A (1975) Le temps mort. Nouvelle Revue de Psychanalyse, 11

Green A (1983) Narcissisme de vie, narcissisme de mort. Editions de Minuit, Paris

Green A (1990) La folie privée. Gallimard, Paris

Grunberger B (1975) Le narcissisme. Payot, Paris

Hitter-Spinelli B (1979) Les hypocondriaques en milieu psychiatrique : diversité nosologique et unité du discours. Medicine Dissertation, Amiens

Israël L (1979) L'hystérique, le sexe et le médecin. Masson, Paris

Jankelevitch V (1977) La mort. Flammarion, Paris

Jaques E (1974) Mort et crise du milieu de la vie. In: Psychanalyse du génie créateur. Dunod, Paris

Journiac A (1888) Recherches cliniques sur le délire hypocondriaque. Dissertation, Paris

Lacan J (1966) Ecrits. Seuil, Paris

Laplanche J (1970) Vie et Mort en psychanalyse. Flammarion, Paris

Leclaire S (1968) Psychanalyser. Seuil, Paris

Leclaire S (1975) On tue un enfant. Seuil, Paris

Levy F (1973) Le malade imaginaire et le médecin malgré lui. Psychologie médicale 5(2):345–357

Loras O (1974) Le monde des entrailles. In: Neurologie psychiatrie. Sandoz, Paris

Marguery G (1949) Les cénestopathies. Dissertation, Toulouse

Marty P (1976) Les mouvements individuels de vie et de mort. Essai d'économie psychosomatique. Payot, Paris

Marty P, de M'Uzan M, David C (1963) L'investigation psychosomatique. P.U.F, Paris

Moliere (Jean-Baptiste Poquelin) Le malade imaginaire. In: Œuvres complètes, Tome II. Gallimard, La Pléiade, Paris

Oules J (1970) Les névroses du troisième âge. Confrontations psychiatriques, 5

Rank O (1922) Le double. French edition: Rank O (1932) (trans: Lautman S). Denoël, Paris

Rank O (1924) Le traumatisme de la naissance. French edition: Rank O (1976) (trans: Lautman S)

Rosenfeld H (1958) Some Psychopathological Observations about Hypocondriacal States. International Journal of Psycho-Analysis, 39

Rosolato G (1975) L'axe narcissique des dépressions. Nouvelle Revue de Psychanalyse, 11

Spielrein S (1981) Entre Freud et Jung. Aubier Montaigne, Paris

Steichen R (1972) La notion de corporéité dans le vécu de l'hypocondriaque. Acta psychiatrica belgica 72(1972):366–381

Timsit M, Dugardin JC, Adam A, Sabatter J (1973) La névrose hypocondriaque a-t-elle droit de cité? Acta psychiatrica belgica. Bruxelles

Valabrega (Jean-Paul) (1954) Les théories psychosomatiques. P.U.F., Paris

Watzlawick et al (1974) Change: Principles of Problem Formation and Problem Resolution. French edition: Watzlawick et al (1975) Changements, paradoxe et psychothérapie. Seuil, Paris

Winnicott DW (1958) Through Paediatrics to Psychoanalysis. Tavistock, London. French edition: Winnicott DW (1969) (trans: Kalmanovitch J). De la pédiatrie à la psychanalyse. Payot, Paris

Winnicott DW (1971) Playing and Reality. Tavistock, London. French edition: Winnicott DW (1975) (trans: Monod C et Pontalis JB). Jeu et réalité. L'espace potentiel. Gallimard, Paris

Winnicott DW (1975) La crainte de l'effondrement. Nouvelle Revue de Psychanalyse, 11

Printed in the United States
By Bookmasters